**INSTRUCTIONAL MANUAL — INDIVIDUAL VERSION**

# Get Fit Gang Fitness Program

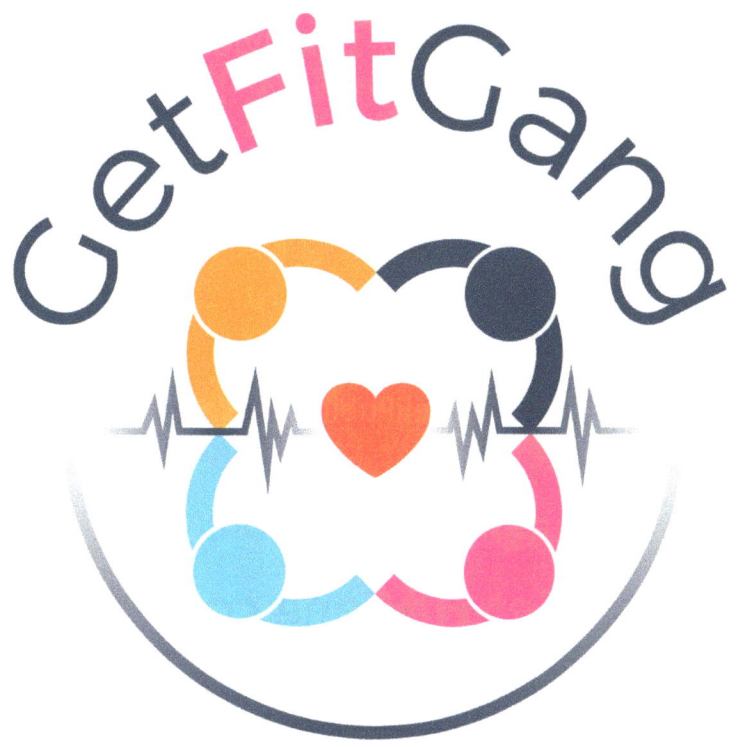

*A 30 minute turn key,
whole body HIIT program made simple!*

©Get Fit Gang, LLC 2020
Katie Wiseman, M.Ed

**INSTRUCTIONAL MANUAL — INDIVIDUAL VERSION**

© Copyright 2020, Katie Wiseman, M.Ed

All rights reserved. No part of this book may be used or reproduced by any means, graphic, electronic, or mechanical, including photocopying, recording, taping or by any information storage retrieval system without the written permission of the publisher except in the case of brief quotations embodied in critical articles and reviews.

ISBN: 978-1-948638-37-1 (INDIVIDUAL EDITION)

Published by:

Fideli Publishing, Inc.
119 W Morgan St.
Martinsville, IN 46151
888-343-3542

www.FideliPublishing.com

For more information, visit:

**Get-Fit-Gang.com**

*Always consult your physician before beginning any exercise program. Consult with your healthcare professional to make sure this is an appropriate exercise prescription for you. If you experience any pain or difficulty with these exercises, stop and consult your healthcare provider.*

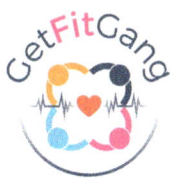

# Acknowledgements

Without the assistance of two very important people, and the most influential person in my life, this project would still be embedded within my mind, as it has been for the past 16 years.

The first is my photographer extraordinaire, Billy Morquecho. After 3 sessions and hundreds of shots, Billy created the series of photos that follow. I hope they will serve to guide you to create clean lines and proper body alignment as you move toward increasing strength and endurance of mind and body (Contact info @billymorquecho).

The second is my confidant, my closest friend and partner in crime, my Irish twin, Nora Cortino. Without her consistent motivation and significant belief in me throughout my life, this book would not have found it's way to these pages.

The last and most influential person in my life is my high school coach, Clyde Wallace. Although he now lives with the angels, he was instrumental in showing me discipline, how to tap into my inner strength, how to work hard and dream big, and what it looked like to live with integrity. I followed him around like a puppy and experienced life through the eyes of someone who profoundly believed in me. It was through those eyes I found the vision of the woman I could become.

Thank you all for helping create this manuscript to help strengthen the bodies of others, so they in turn can successfully impact the lives of those they love.

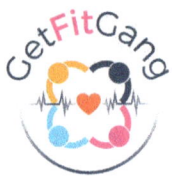

# Preface

Ever thought about joining a gang? If not, I'd like you to rethink that one.

I know of a gang that focuses on self-care, self-esteem and strength.

A gang that helps build confidence, mental clarity and nurtures pride.

A gang where being a member fosters resilience and promotes mental health and well-being.

The longer you're a member the stronger you become.

Being a part of this gang is actually good for you!

It helps improve sleep, digestion, alertness, stamina and happiness.

Being a part of this gang can make a world of difference!

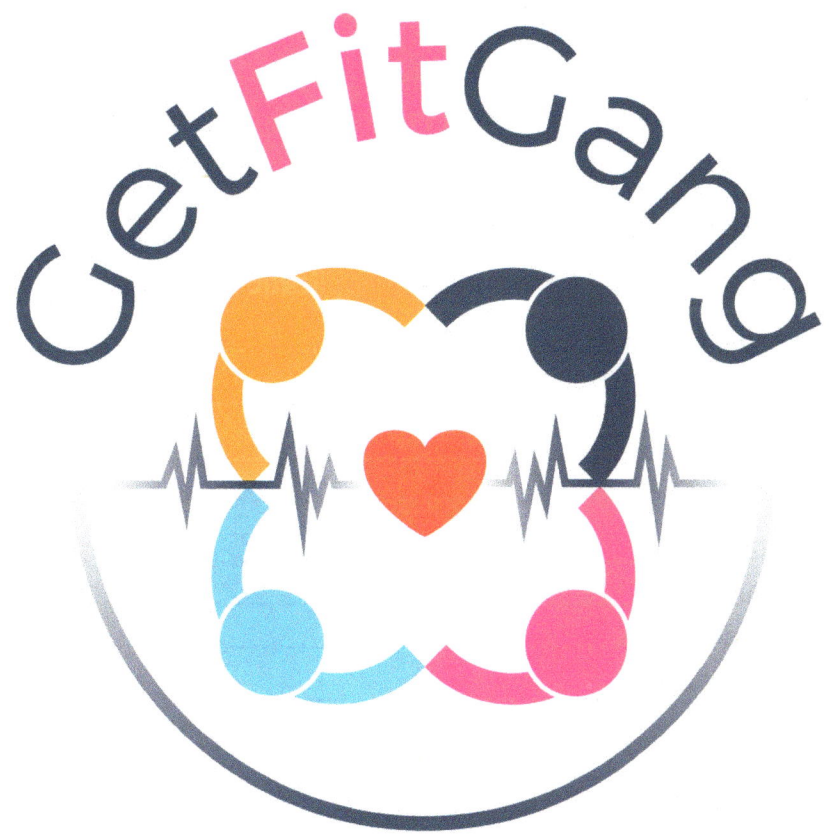

# Table of Contents

©Get Fit Gang, LLC 2020
Katie Wiseman

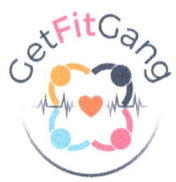

# Table of Contents

| | | |
|---|---|---|
| I. | Introduction | 9 |
| II. | Elements of the Get Fit Gang Fitness Program | 17 |
| III. | How to Conduct Program | 21 |
| IV. | Benefits of the Get Fit Gang Fitness Program | 23 |
| V. | Instructional Guide - Demonstration and application of techniques and skills | 29 |

- <u>Standard Tasks</u> ................................................ 30
- Push Up ............................................................ 31
- Straight Leg ...................................................... 33
  - I. Bend Knee ................................................. 33
- Abdominals ....................................................... 34
  - I. Curl ............................................................ 34
  - II. Scissor Legs ............................................. 37
- Forearm Plank ................................................... 40
- Bridge w/Band .................................................. 42
- Straight Arm Plank ........................................... 45
- Shoulder Raises ................................................ 48
  - I. Front Raises .............................................. 50
  - II. Lateral Raises .......................................... 50
- Upper-Mid Back ................................................. 51
  - I. Reverse Flys ............................................. 51
  - II. Scarecrow ................................................ 54
- Triceps Kickback ............................................... 57
- Lunges .............................................................. 60
- Squats .............................................................. 63
- Step Series ....................................................... 66

©Get Fit Gang, LLC 2020
Katie Wiseman

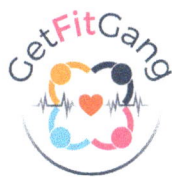

# Table of Contents (CONTINUED)

- ➢ **Modified Tasks** .................................................................. 70
    - Push Up .................................................................. 71
        - I. Push Up at Wall .......................................... 73
    - Abdominals ............................................................. 74
        - I. Curl .......................................................... 74
        - II. Scissor Legs ............................................. 77
    - Forearm Plank ......................................................... 80
    - Bridge without band ................................................ 82
    - Straight Arm Plank .................................................. 84
    - Shoulder Raises ....................................................... 87
        - I. Front Raises ............................................. 89
        - II. Lateral Raises .......................................... 89
    - Upper-Mid Back ...................................................... 90
        - I. Reverse Flys ............................................. 90
        - II. Scarecrow ................................................ 93
    - Triceps Kickback ..................................................... 96
    - Lunge at steps ......................................................... 99
    - Squats at wall w/ball ............................................... 102

VI. Time Chart ........................................................................ 105
VII. Get Fit Gang Supplies ....................................................... 107
VIII. Get Fit Gang Tracker Form ............................................... 113
IX. Contact Information .......................................................... 116
X. 2-Part Exercise Station Poster ............................................ 119

©Get Fit Gang, LLC 2020
Katie Wiseman

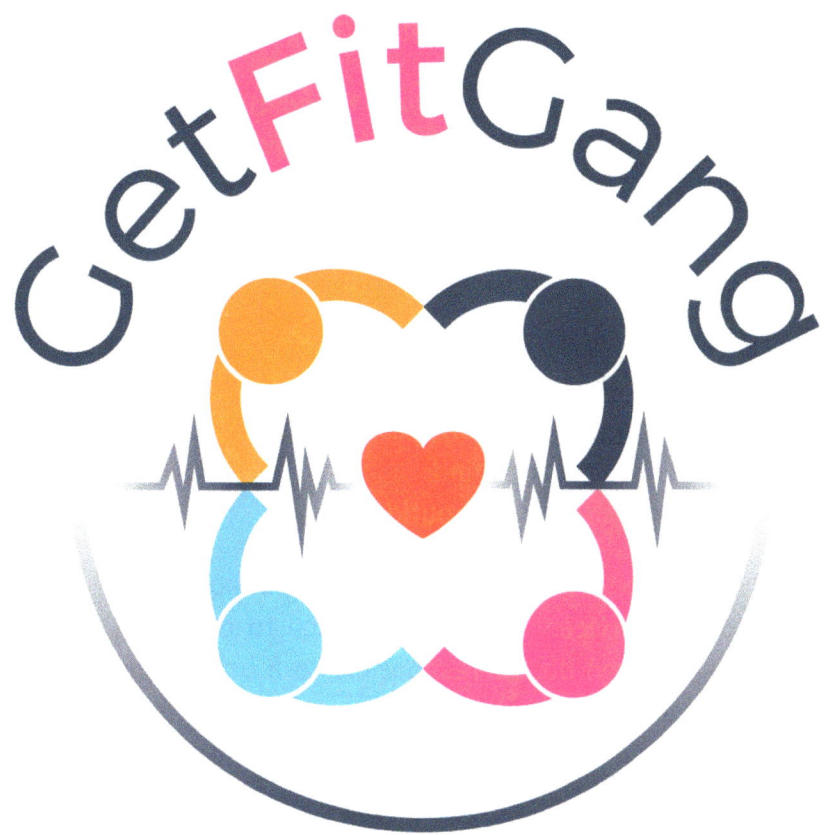

# Introduction

©Get Fit Gang, LLC 2020
Katie Wiseman

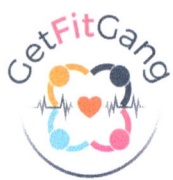

# Introduction

Congratulations on your purchase of the Get Fit Gang fitness program!

Your commitment to this program will lay a foundation of strength, endurance and overall physical and emotional wellness. The body craves strength!

Strong bodies:

- Keep stress at bay
- Enjoy hardy immune systems
- Profit from deep sleep at night
- Provide increased energy, stamina and resiliency
- Recognize clarity of thought and mind
- And, generally have a more positive outlook on life

I chose the field of public service because it is my passion, my gift to the world. We really are all people in service. We are in service to others as parents, employees, husbands and wives, or even bosses responsible to a board, humans are continuously pouring out the best of themselves in service, as it should be to live vibrant lives. However, when we give most of our strength to others, it leaves a deficit and many of us struggle to find a way to fill the void. Interestingly, what fills the void is strength, earned and given once again. This is the cycle of a healthy lifestyle, but often many people are stuck in just the giving part and not the earing back part.

The Get Fit Gang fitness program hopes to replenish the deficit by providing a turn-key, whole body fitness program that's easy to follow and easy to implement, whereby the body can earn strength and stamina and more easily find the balance required to stay healthy and refreshed. As odd as it may sound, the body is most happy when it feels strong and able to meet challenges with ease.

The Get Fit Gang fitness program is a HIIT (High Intensity Interval Training) program and is designed to help you gain physical strength, increase cardiovascular endurance and provides an outlet to flush toxins, all in a 30 minute time frame in the comfort of your own home or personal gym setting.

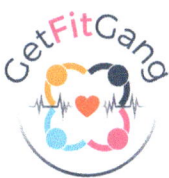

# Introduction

The Get Fit Gang fitness program is designed to help you gain physical strength, increase cardiovascular endurance, and provides an outlet to flush toxins, all in a 30 minute time frame within the comfort of your own home.

As a collegiate athlete I know the importance of a strong body. I am also a single mom of four and like many of you, I found it too difficult to find the time to move my body to earn strength. Just getting out of bed on some days felt like a victory. But, the lack of vigorous activity caught up to me. I realized I was 40 pounds overweight, felt sluggish and tired most of the time and hated the way my body looked and felt in clothes. I decided it was time to earn back the strength I so coveted in my college days.

As a collegiate athlete, I know the importance of a strong body. I am also a single mom of four, and like many of you I found it too difficult to find time to move my body, so I didn't...for years! One day, I was so disgusted with the way I felt, the way my clothes fit and the sluggishness I experienced everywhere in my body, that I decided enough is enough!

Although I missed what a strong body provides and longed for a physical outlet, I still didn't know where I could fit in a workout with regularity. I needed something effective, but quick. Some way to earn lasting strength, but that didn't take long. I needed something easy to follow and easy to complete, but it had to give the rigor required to earn strength.

I turned to my expertise (my degree is in Health and Physical Education) and deep down I realized the answer! The strategy my coaches used along the way if they had little or no time to spare, **_high intensity interval training_** is the way to go. Intense bursts of movement, followed by brief moments of rest. This is the best way to get the biggest bang for your buck in the smallest amount of time. This was the answer! It was 2002 when I decided to launch the first Get Fit Gang fitness program on my elementary school campus.

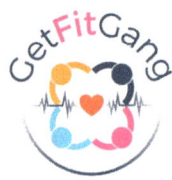

# Introduction

The program has evolved over the past 16 years as I have tweaked some elements and refined the system to become more efficient all while maintaining ease of implementation requiring minimal space and equipment. The Get Fit Gang fitness program individual version is designed for busy people who need a quick, but effective exercise program to gain strength and endurance in the quickest possible amount of time. The Get Fit Gang fitness program is a HIIT program that integrates both strength and cardio into a research based exercise regimen that provides the possibility to gain strength and cardiovascular endurance in an intense but highly effective program that gets quick results.

The program is designed to target all major muscle groups, including the heart and lungs. It builds strength and endurance through interval training…moments of high intensity work (not to be confused with high impact) followed with brief amounts of recovery time.

In the Get Fit Gang fitness program, you complete 10 strength training exercises (tasks) interspersed with 6 cardiovascular tasks (steps). This program is designed to target all major muscle groups, including thighs, hamstrings, glutes, abdominals, shoulders, back, triceps and most importantly the heart and lungs.

Each exercise session begins with a 90 second step interval to elevate the cardiovascular system and to light the fire within. After 90 seconds on the steps, there is a brief 30 second transition period, where participants go to the first of 10 strength conditioning exercises. Each task will be completed for 90 seconds, followed by another 30 second transition period.

After the completion of 2 strength training tasks, there is a transition back to the steps for another cardiovascular series on the steps. This cycle repeats until all 10 strength tasks and 6 series of steps have been completed (total time 31:30).

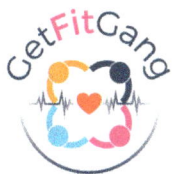

# Introduction

Your mindset during this program is vital to your success. Setting yourself up to work with high intensity for each of the 90 second intervals is valuable beyond what is usually expected. Challenging yourself physically is of course always beneficial, you will gain strength, which raises your metabolism, increases energy and will elevate your mood (think happy endorphins emoji here!). It also provides an opportunity to flush toxins and combat negativity, which can often consume our thoughts after a particularly challenging day.

Recognizing this as an opportunity to challenge your mind is equally beneficial and often overlooked. Engaging in just 30 minutes of exercise on a regular basis helps boost your memory, improves concentration and can enhance your overall mental and emotional health and well-being, especially over time.

I trust you feel inspired and are realizing the benefits of the program and are prepared to buy and become a Get Fit Gang gangster. But there is one more important matter that needs to be shared. It may come as a shock to you, it did to me, but current research confirms the following statement.

**Lack of exercise is killing us! Inactivity is worse for you than smoking and diabetes!**

The most current scientific research of a 23 year study following 122,000 people confirms that lack of exercise is worse for your health than smoking or diabetes! This startling research, which was published in 2018 prompted me to finally get this program on paper and to share with others.

Knowing how busy our lives are, and how difficult it can be to find time to schedule exercise should not limit us from making a commitment to move our bodies. Movement needs to be intentional in everyone's life. Gaining strength needs to be a priority in our lives. Strong bodies are happy bodies and happy bodies prosper!

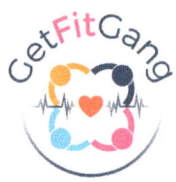

## Introduction

Moving our bodies is essential to quality of life. Participating in the Get Fit Gang fitness program can be an effective way to increase strength and endurance, but will also provide opportunities to nurture you mind, offset the harmful effects of stress, boost your immune system and help you enjoy your life with a new sense of vitality that only strength of body and mind can endorse. It time to envision a stronger you! Let the Get Fit Gang fitness program help you realize your absolute best self!

**You picked a great time to get started! Let's get this done!**

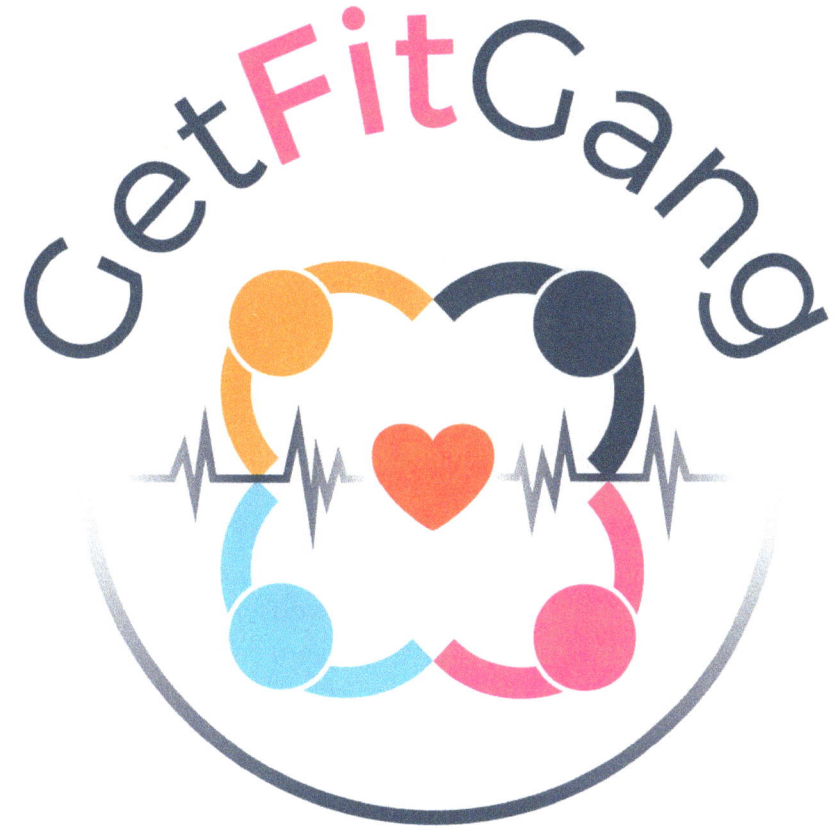

# Elements of the Get Fit Gang Group Fitness Program

©Get Fit Gang, LLC 2020
Katie Wiseman

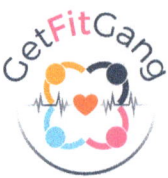

# Elements of the Get Fit Gang Fitness Program

**Main Objectives:**

- Elevation of heart rate, which is critical to increase stamina and gain strength.

- Gaining strength, which will boost overall body functions (sleep, digestion, etc.), promote confidence and clarity of thought, increase energy, stamina and overall emotional health and well-being.

- Increasing cardiovascular strength and endurance.

- Striving for perfect body alignment during movement by focusing on key elements during tasks (instructional guide included) which will expedite gains in both strength and endurance.

- Safety during movement by correct body alignment to ensure no pain in any joint at any time. If you experience discomfort in a joint your body is telling you something is wrong, and a modification MUST occur to prevent injury. (Note: the Get Fit Gang fitness program includes modifications for each task).

- Intention to set small goals or "tweak" intensity with each workout session to continue to grow in strength and endurance and boost metabolic rate for up to 36 hours after exercise!

**Benefits:**

- Increased Strength
- Increased Metabolism
- Increased Stamina
- Increased Heart/Lung Capacity
- Increased Clarity and Mental Alertness
- Reduced Levels of Stress

©Get Fit Gang, LLC 2020
Katie Wiseman

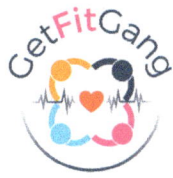

# Elements of the Get Fit Gang Fitness Program

**Materials:  (Reference materials information on page 107)**

- Music

- Aerobic steps (or mini trampoline)

- Thick individual yoga mat

- (1)  6" - 8" yoga or playground balls for use with the Abdominals, Forearm Plank, Straight Arm Plank and modified Bridge w/Ball stations

- (1) 10"- 12" playground ball to use for modified squat at wall (if needed for modification)

- Exercise band for glutes station

- 1 - 2 sets of Heavy weights (6 - 15 lb.) mid-range for Flys and heavier for Lunges/Squats

- 1 set of Light weights (2 - 5 lb.)

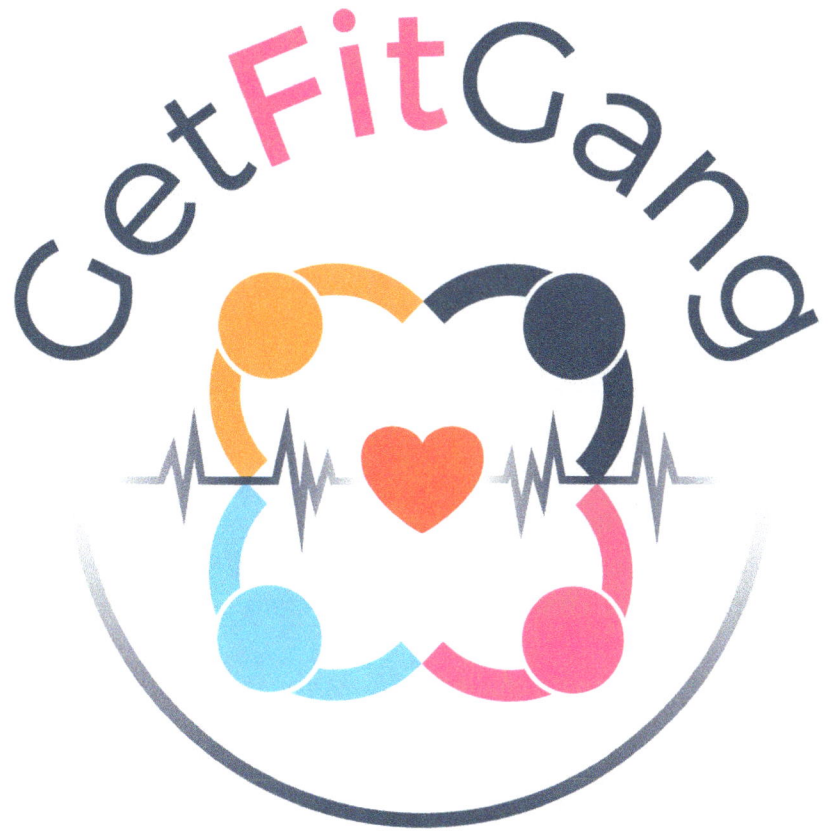

# How to Conduct the Program

©Get Fit Gang, LLC 2020
Katie Wiseman

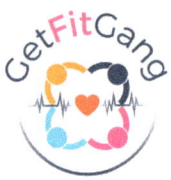

# How to Conduct the Program

1. Set up materials and music. (For a the full list of the equipment refer to page 107) Make sure to keep props out of the way to ensure lanes for safe movement.

2. Set up means to transition. You may use Get Fit Gang audio, stop watch, clock or your phone.

3. Using the laminated time and task chart (included) start the program on the steps.

4. Complete each of the tasks for 90 seconds. Pay close attention to the half way mark during Station 2, Abdominals; Station 6, Shoulders Raises; and Station 7 Reverse Fly, as you change tasks at 45 seconds.

5. Pay close attention to the number of repetitions you are able to accomplish during each task. This will not only help keep your mind off fatigue, but will help you gage your improvement as you continue with the program.

6. After completing **two** strength challenge tasks, you will transition back to the steps (or mini trampoline) for another cardio series.

7. After all 10 strength challenge tasks have been completed, finish the program with one last 90 second step series. Time required 31:30.

8. A brief stretch after the program is highly recommended. Check out the website for a quick stretch series.

9. Ideally complete the program three times per week.

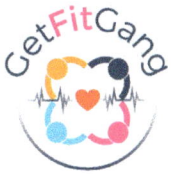

# How to Conduct the Program

10. A brief stretch after the program is highly encouraged.

To simplify, the program looks like this:

- Steps
- Strength challenge Task 1 and 2
- Steps
- Strength challenge Task 3 and 4
- Steps
- Strength challenge Task 5 and 6
- Steps
- Strength challenge Task 7 and 8
- Steps
- Strength challenge Task 9 and 10
- Steps

Total Time: 31:30

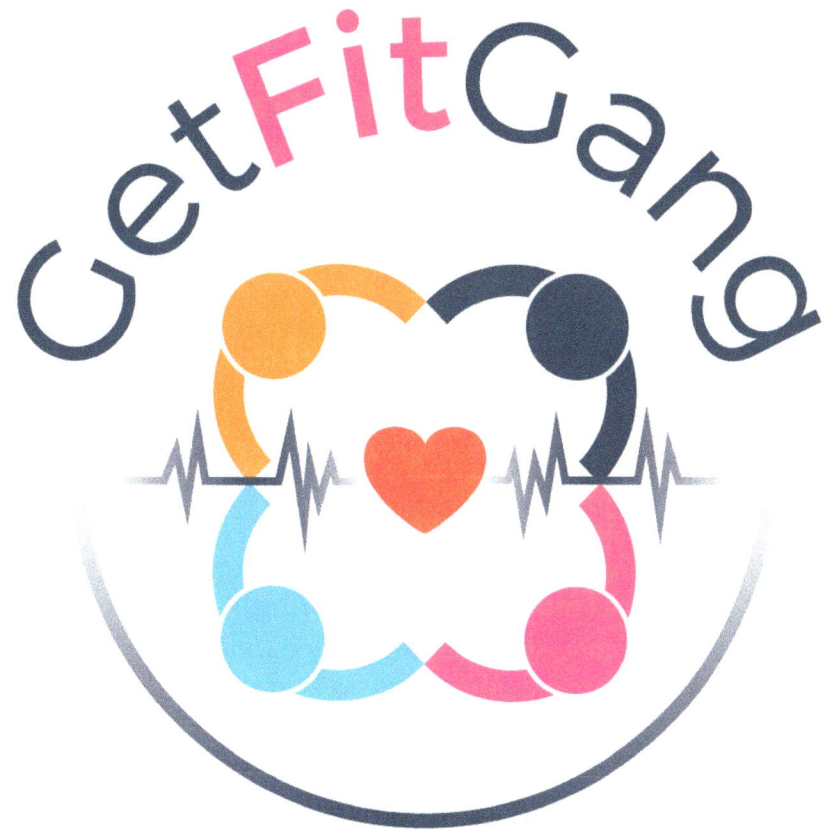

# Benefits of the Get Fit Gang Fitness Program

©Get Fit Gang, LLC 2020
Katie Wiseman

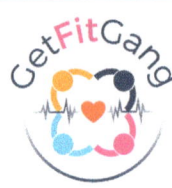

## Exercise Benefits

| Exercise | Benefits | Example |
|---|---|---|
| Push Ups<br>Bent Knee<br>Or<br>Straight Leg | Targets pectoral muscles (chest)<br><br>Targets triceps (back of the arm)<br><br>Targets shoulders<br><br>Strengthens abdominals<br><br>Strengthens back side of body | |
| **TOTAL BODY STRENGTHENER** | | |
| Abdominal Curl<br>Scissor Leg | Extremely important muscle group; regardless of the motion, all movement ripples through the core; stabilizes the body during movement.<br><br>Weak or inflexible abdominals impair how your body functions during any movement.<br><br>Improves everyday tasks;<br><br>Creates balance in the body.<br><br>Improves the function of the lower back by providing support.<br><br>Improves balance, stability and posture. | |
| **CORE STRENGTH** | | |

©Get Fit Gang, LLC 2020
Katie Wiseman

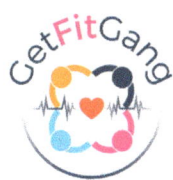

| Exercise | Benefits | Example |
|---|---|---|
| Forearm Plank | Full body workout – abdominals back, hips, legs, shoulders, chest<br><br>Targets abdominals<br><br>Improves posture<br><br>Improves mental ability<br><br>Stabilizes the spine | |
| **TOTAL BODY STRENGTHENER** | | |
| Bridge with Band | Assists with a strong posture.<br><br>Can decrease knee pain due to lack of strength (control) of the upper leg at the hip joint.<br><br>Safely works the posterior muscles including the glutes, hamstrings and lower back.<br><br>Strengthens your core, especially your transverse (lower) abdominals.<br><br>Improved strength can eliminate pressure on the lower back. | |
| **GLUTES** | | |

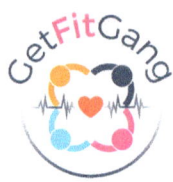

| Exercise | Benefits | Example |
|---|---|---|
| Straight Arm Plank | Full body workout — abdominals back, hips, legs, shoulders, chest<br><br>Targets abdominals<br><br>Improves posture<br><br>Stabilizes the spine | |
| **TOTAL BODY STRENGTHENER** | | |
| Front/Lateral Shoulder Raises | Targets the deltoids promoting strength and stability of the entire shoulder girdle.<br><br>Core is involved to stabilize the movement.<br><br>Shoulder strength will increase performance in all exercises using the shoulder, such as planks. | |
| **SHOULDER GIRDLE** | | |

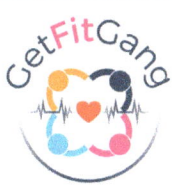

| Exercise | Benefits | Example |
|---|---|---|
| Reverse Flys Scarecrow | Strengthens the posterior shoulder and upper back.<br><br>Improves body posture.<br><br>Targets upper back muscles creating more length on the front side of the body. | |
| **UPPER/MID BACK** | | |
| Triceps Kickbacks | Helps stabilize the shoulder joint.<br><br>Increases functionality, flexibility and range of motion of arm movements.<br><br>Largest muscle group in the upper arm responsible for lower arm extension. | |
| **UPPER ARM** | | |

Exercise Benefits

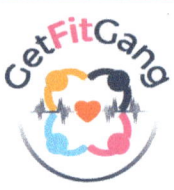

| Exercise | Benefits | Example |
|---|---|---|
| Lunge:<br><br>Or<br><br>Modified Lunge w/Weights | Targets core stability<br><br>Develops better balance<br><br>Strengthens legs and glutes<br><br>Improves hip flexibility<br><br>Improves the health of the spine | |
| **TOTAL BODY STRENGTHENER** | | |
| Squat:<br><br>With Weights<br><br>Or<br><br>Without Weights<br><br>Or<br><br>With Weights at Wall (with ball) | Intensive full body movement<br><br>Targets all major muscle groups (Glutes, abdominals, quads, hamstrings, calves).<br><br>Increases muscle growth thereby increasing metabolism.<br><br>Improves the pumping of fluids throughout the body by engaging the largest muscle groups of the body.<br><br>Improves transfer of nutrients and elimination of toxins. | |
| **TOTAL BODY STRENGTHENER** | | |

Exercise Benefits

©Get Fit Gang, LLC 2020
Katie Wiseman

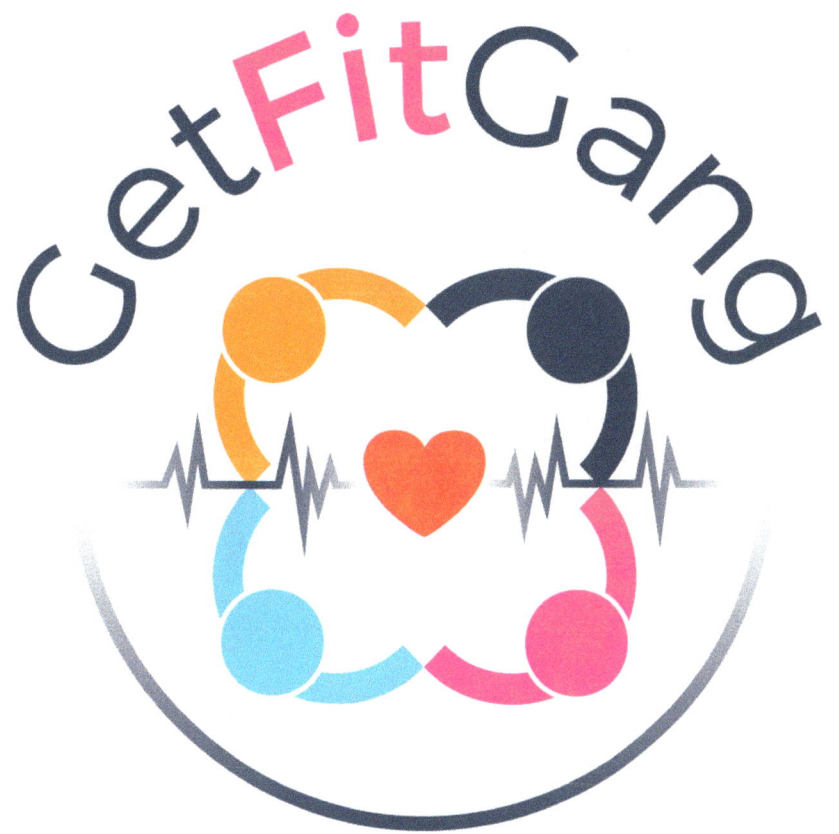

# Instructional Guide
# Standard Tasks

©Get Fit Gang, LLC 2020
Katie Wiseman

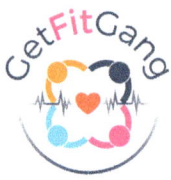

# Instructional Guide – Standard Tasks

Instructional Guide – Demonstration and application of techniques and skills.

Standard Tasks ............................................................................................ 30
- Push Up .......................................................................................... 31
    - I. Straight Leg ........................................................................... 31
    - II. Bend Knee ............................................................................ 31

- Abdominals ................................................................................... 34
    - I. Curl ........................................................................................ 34
    - II. Scissor Legs .......................................................................... 37

- Forearm Plank .............................................................................. 40

- Bridge w/Band .............................................................................. 42

- Straight Arm Plank ....................................................................... 45

- Shoulder Raises ............................................................................ 48
    - I. Front Raises .......................................................................... 48
    - II. Lateral Raises ....................................................................... 48

- Upper-Mid Back ........................................................................... 51
    - I. Reverse Fly ............................................................................ 51
    - II. Scarecrow ............................................................................ 54

- Triceps Kickback .......................................................................... 57

- Lunges .......................................................................................... 60

- Squats ........................................................................................... 63

- Step Series ................................................................................... 66

©Get Fit Gang, LLC 2020
Katie Wiseman

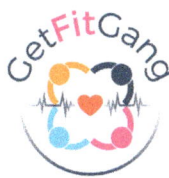

## **Standard Push Ups**

**Total Body Strengthener**

**(Most gang members will use the bent knee format until adequate strength is acquired to ensure correct body alignment when using straight leg format).**

**Set-Up:**

- On the mat, knees are bent, with feet reaching toward glutes.

- Avoid placing body weight directly on knee caps. Try instead to be on the meaty part of the thigh above the knee.

- Hands are placed off the mat, wider than shoulder width, but within the same lateral plane as the shoulders. Place entire hand onto the floor, opening the fingers by extending the webbing between the fingers and placing all knuckles on the floor, especially the index finger and thumb to help protect the wrists.

- Abdominals are engaged by slightly tipping the tailbone down and away, elongating the lower back and hollowing out the core.

- Eyes gaze is slightly forward of the fingers.

**Movement:**

- Think of the movement as a moving plank…the entire body "form" moves down and up, not just chest, or chin.

- Lead with the sternum (chest) by bending the elbows, keeping core engaged and lower as far as possible without collapsing either the abdominals or shoulders (Note: only go deep enough to keep strict form…as strength is gained, depth will increase).

- Inhale as the body moves down and exhale forcefully as the body returns…fill up and release each time….breathing is fuel for your body during movement, so to ensure your body can stay engaged throughout the 90 second interval, breathe with fluidity. Extend arms fully at the top of the movement, but elbows remain soft.

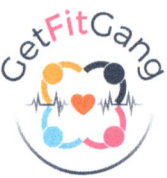

- If possible, catch the beat of the music and move with the rhythm of the beat.

- Move as controlled as possible…don't rush through the movement. Slow and steady gets the job done. Core engagement is the key to success! Slight tilt of the tailbone down and away as you hollow out the core to elongate the lower back.

- Continue, focusing on body alignment, breath and a deep contraction of abdominal muscles throughout the timed task.

- Keep track from one session to the next on how many repetitions you are able to accomplish. This will serve as your goal and provide incentive to grow in strength and endurance throughout the year.

- Option: Place a ball high between the upper thighs to provide stability to the hips, engage the lower abdominals, inner thighs and to provide a slight inner rotation of the femur bone so knees maintain strict alignment.

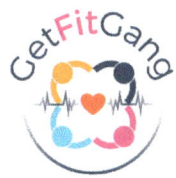

## Bent-Knee

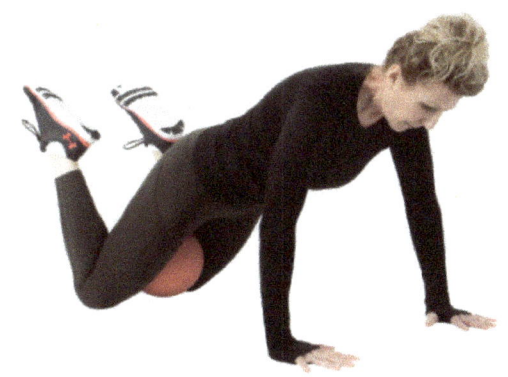  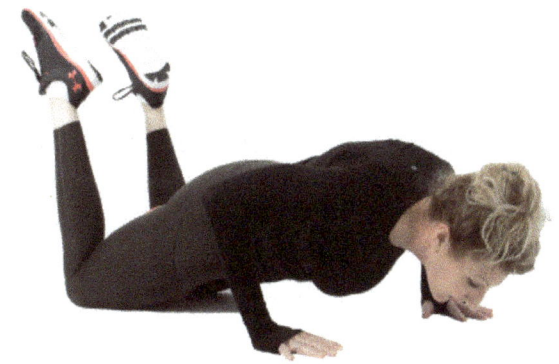

**START**　　　　　　　　　　　**END**

## Straight Leg

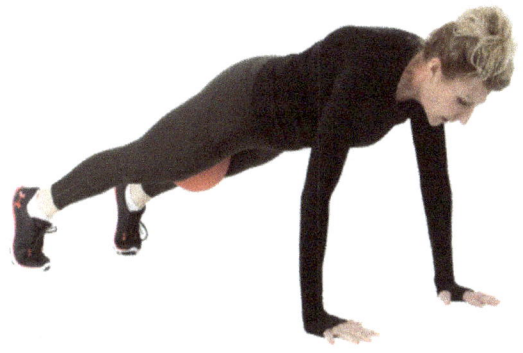  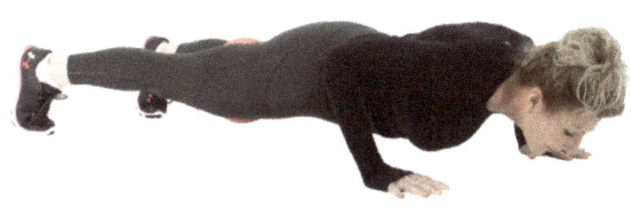

**START**　　　　　　　　　　　**END**

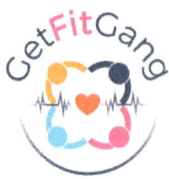

**Standard Abdominal Curl** – Complete for the first 45 seconds of the task.

**Set-Up:**

- Lay on mat, facing up, knees are bent with sacrum (flat bone at the base of the spine) in contact with the mat and feet flat on the floor.

- Place hands behind your head and rest head in hands. Keep elbows wide (like a pillow)! You don't want to see your elbows in your peripheral vision.

- Visualize an apple between your chin and chest. Try to prevent dropping chin toward your chest, so the abdominals are doing the work, not the neck.

**Movement:**

- Visualize drilling the navel to the spine to begin the movement, then lift the shoulder blades as high off the mat as possible reaching the chest (sternum) toward the ceiling, exhaling to maintain tight abdominals at the top of the range of movement and without dropping the chin toward the chest. Tilt the hip bones toward shoulders slightly as you reach the top of the range of movement, which will ground the lower back further into the mat.

- The elbows stay wide, head rests in hands, as you lift the chest (sternum) straight up toward the ceiling.

- Exhale as you lift the shoulders, engage the core and inhale as you return to the mat.

- Breathing pattern is critical to keep abdominals contracting and expanding in the correct sequence.

- Pause briefly at the top of the range of movement as you deflate the lungs, tipping the hips toward the shoulders, which will push the abdominals even further into the mat.

- Make a mental connection between your body and mind throughout the movement. This focus will help deepen the muscular engagement and help regulate your breath.

- Range of movement is not large; you are lifting just the shoulder blades off the mat, reaching the sternum toward the ceiling. A burning sensation will be felt in the upper abdominals fairly quickly when movement and breath coordinate.

©Get Fit Gang, LLC 2020
Katie Wiseman

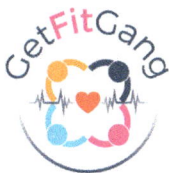

- Try not to rush through the movement and focus on your breath. Quality of movement, especially with mental focus wins over quantity.

- Continue, focusing on body alignment, breath and a deep contraction of abdominal muscles throughout the timed task.

- Keep track from one class to the next how many repetitions you are able to accomplish. This will serve as your goal and provide incentive to grow in strength and endurance throughout the year.

- Option: Place a ball high between the upper thighs to provide stability to the hips, engage the lower abdominal, inner thighs and to provide a slight inner rotation of the femur bone so knees maintain strict alignment.

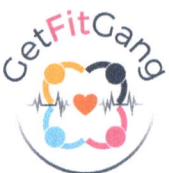

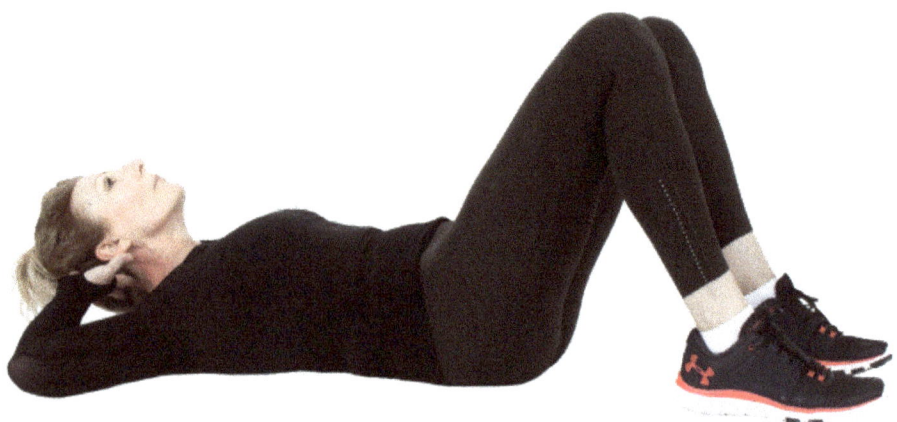

**START**

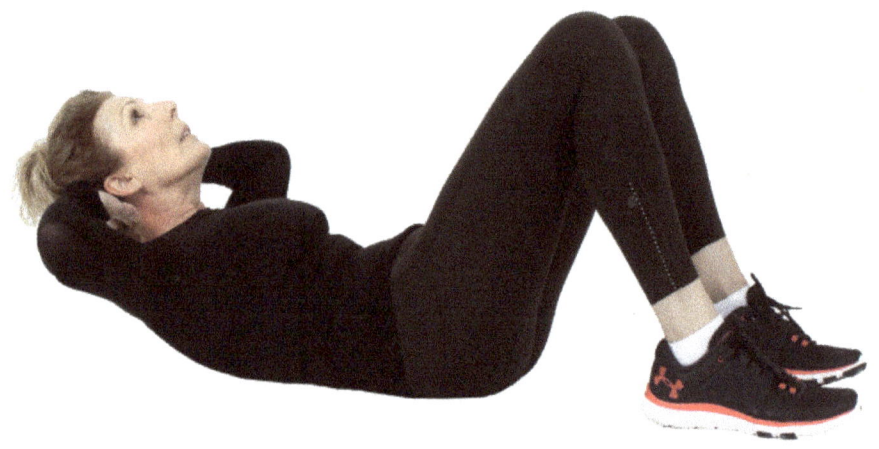

**END**

©Get Fit Gang, LLC 2020
Katie Wiseman

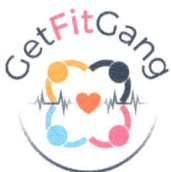

### Standard Abdominal Scissor Legs

Complete for the second 45 seconds of the task.

**Set-Up:**

- Lay down on back and extend legs into the air directly above the hips.

- Place hands under sacrum (flat bone located at the base of the spine) for support.

- Rest head on mat.

- Engage abdominals, by tilting hipbones toward shoulders and hollowing out core.

- Slight bend in the knee to keep movement in the lower abdominals and out of the hip flexors.

- Point toes toward ceiling.

**Movement:**

- Initiate movement by engaging abdominals and visualize drilling the navel to the spine. This slight movement will flatten the lower back out even more and engage the deep transverse abdominals.

- Lower one leg at a time as far as possible without touching the ground or allowing the lower back to arch or rise off the mat.

- Exhale as you bring the leg back from the bottom of the range of movement and re-engage the abdominals to raise the leg back to the starting position.

- Repeat series using the other leg.

- Raise the head, neck and shoulders, if possible, to deepen engagement of abdominal wall, but make sure your not straining your neck muscles.

- Focus on rhythmic breathing throughout the movement.

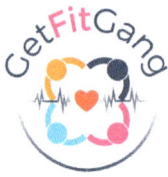

- Control of movement is important…don't just let the leg drop allowing gravity to do the work. Use the core muscles to control the full range of movement, throughout.

- Continue, focusing on body alignment, breath and a deep contraction of abdominal muscles throughout the timed task.

- Keep track from one class to the next how many repetitions you are able to accomplish. This will serve as your goal and provide incentive to grow in strength and endurance throughout the year.

- Option: Place a ball high between the upper thighs to provide stability to the hips, engage the lower abdominals, inner thighs and to provide a slight inner rotation of the femur bone so knees maintain strict alignment.

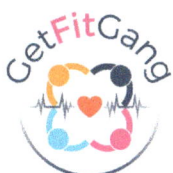

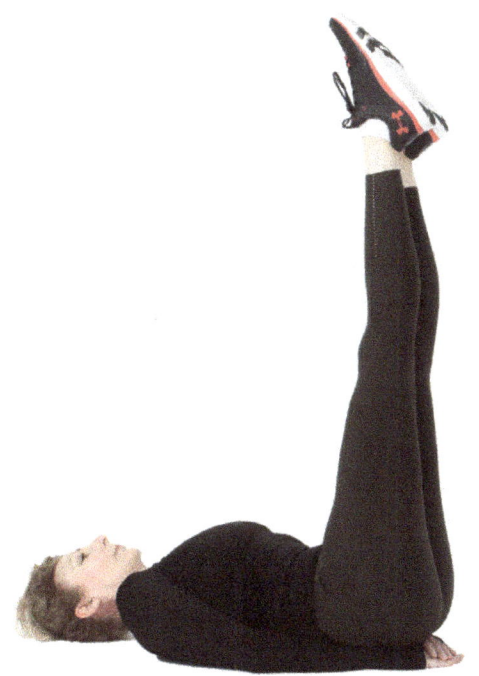

**START**

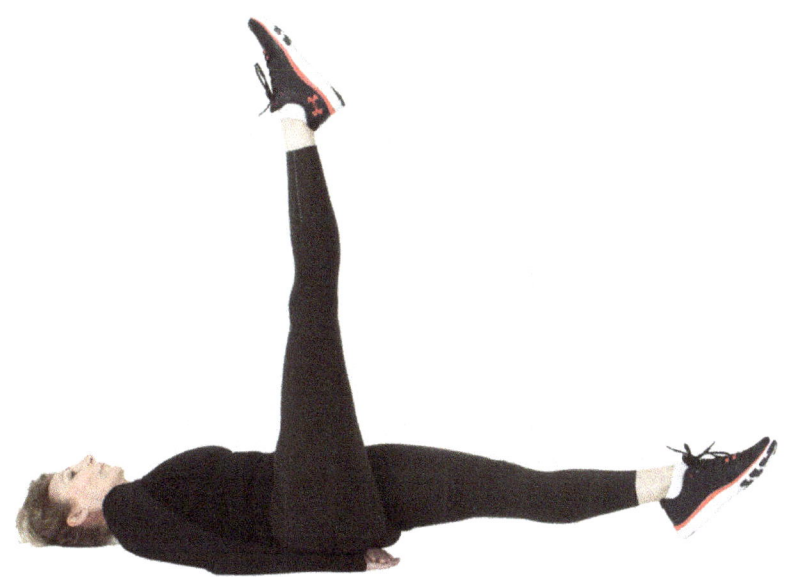

**END**

©Get Fit Gang, LLC 2020
Katie Wiseman

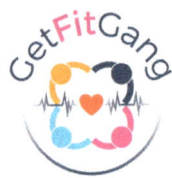

### **Standard Forearm Plank:** Total body strengthener

**Set-Up:** There is no movement with this task.

- Place elbows on mat creating the number eleven (train track) with elbows slightly inside the vertical plane of the shoulders.

- Extend the legs behind you lifting the knees off the mat by engaging the abdominals. Your abdominals serve as a "wall" to support your lower spine. Abdominal engagement is key to the exercise.

- Place entire forearm and entire hand, including finger pads and joints firmly on the mat.

- Come up high on the toes to ensure shoulders are stacked directly over the elbows. Do not allow the shoulders to fall behind the elbows. Strict form allows you to recruit multiple muscle groups to get the most out of the plank.

- Focus on "puffing up" the upper back by stretching out the shoulder blades and rounding the shoulders. Tighten the quadriceps and keep core engaged. This will provide a study base.

- Lift the hips to align with shoulders.

- Abdominals are tight. Think of tipping the tailbone slightly down and away by hollowing out the abdominal wall and drilling the navel to the spine.

- Eyes gaze is slightly up and between the hands, chin points toward floor.

- Breath is your fuel. Maintain this still and silent position for the duration of the 90 seconds.

- This is the most difficult task in the entire series for me. This is an isometric contraction of the muscular system (working muscles without movement at a joint) and a highly effective strength builder. If you must rest, drop knees to mat and return to position as quickly as possible.

- Continue, focusing on body alignment, arching upper back, shoulders over wrists, breath and a deep contraction of abdominal muscles throughout the timed task.

- Option: Place a ball high between the upper thighs to engage the lower abdominals, inner thighs and to provide stability of the hips and a slight inner rotation of the femur bone, knees caps look straight toward floor.

©Get Fit Gang, LLC 2020
Katie Wiseman

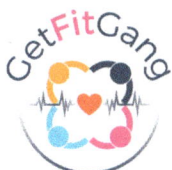
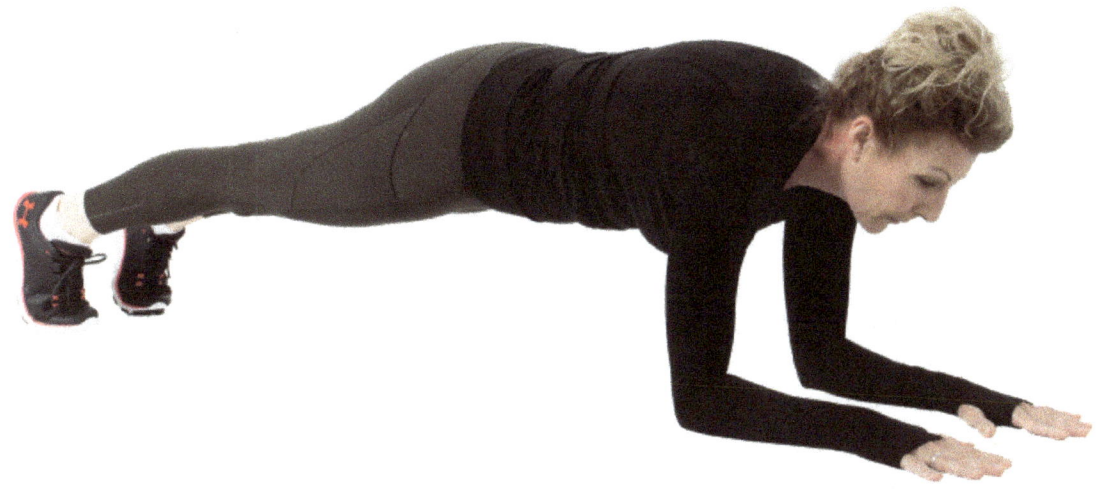

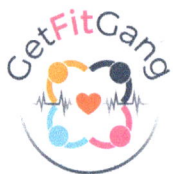

## **Standard Bridge with Band:** Glute Maximus and Medius

**Set-Up:**

- Place resistance band directly above the knees.
- Lay down on the mat on your back, resting your head on the mat with arms resting at the sides of the body.
- Bend your knees and place your feet hip width apart off the mat and onto the floor.

**Movement:**

- Movement is initiated when you engage the abdominal wall by pressing navel to spine, flattening your back against the mat and hollowing out the core by slightly tipping your hip bones forward toward shoulders.
- Dig you heels into the floor as you lift your hips, keeping knees in vertical alignment with hip joint.
- With core tightly engaged, lift the hips as high as you can while keeping mid back and shoulders on the mat.
- At the top of the range of motion, maintaining contact with the mid back and shoulders on the mat, slightly extend knees out by pressing against the resistance band. The range of motion is small and controlled but will engage the outer thighs and glute medius.
- The movement occurs in four counts, with control. Try not to chop the movement, just think of the four components as Up, Out, In, Down…all while keeping core tightly engaged.
- Consciously squeeze the glutes at the top of the range of motion and while extending knees out. This mental engagement will keep the focus on the glutes which are the strongest muscle in the body and need a lot of attention to transform. It also plays a major role in elevating the metabolism, so keep focused!
- Inhale to initiate the movement, exhale at the top of the range of movement and inhale on the way back down to the mat but try not to rest the hips at the bottom of the range of movement. Keep those strong glutes engaged.

©Get Fit Gang, LLC 2020
Katie Wiseman

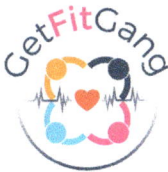

- Continue, focusing on body alignment, breath and a deep contraction of abdominal muscle and glute muscles throughout the timed task.

- Keep track from one class to the next how many repetitions you are able to accomplish. This will serve as your goal and provide incentive to grow in strength and endurance throughout the year.

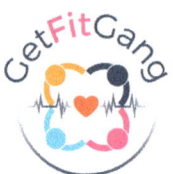

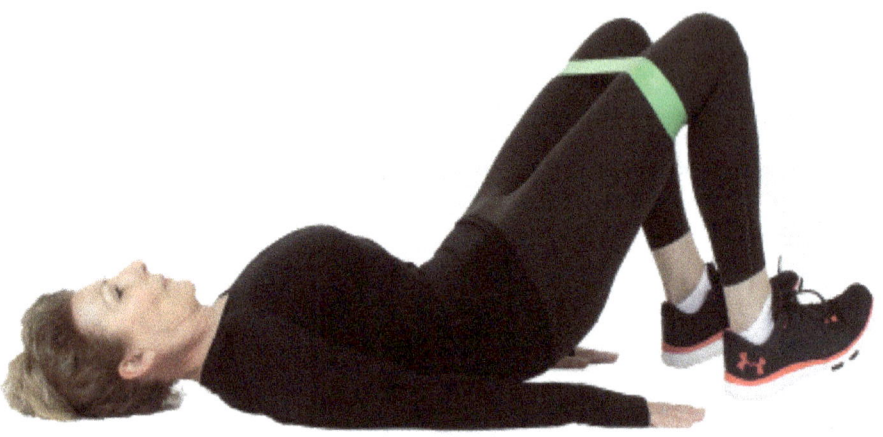

**START**

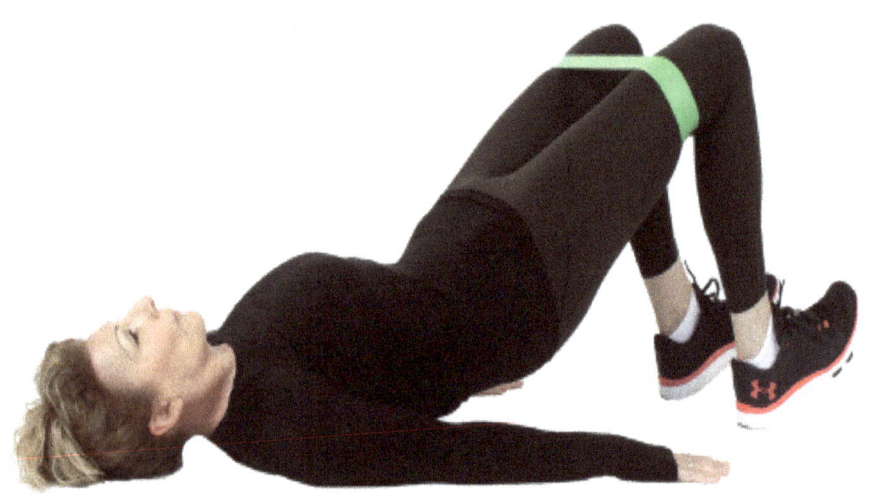

**END**

©Get Fit Gang, LLC 2020
Katie Wiseman

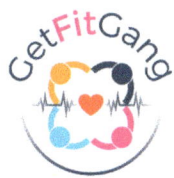

### **Standard Straight Arm Plank:** TOTAL body strengthener

**Set-Up:** There is no movement with this task.

- This task will be done on floor with no mat.

- Place hands on the floor and stack the shoulders directly over the wrists.

- Place entire hand, including finger pads and joints firmly on the floor. Be sure to expand the webbing of the hand and press squarely into the floor with both hands equally.

- Extend the legs behind you by lifting the knees, engage the abdominals and contract your quadriceps (large muscle on the front of the leg).

- Your abdominals serve as a "wall" to support your spine. Tight abdominal engagement is key to the exercise.

- Come up as high as possible on the balls of the feet and push hips forward to ensure shoulders are stacked directly over the wrists. Do not allow the shoulders to fall behind the wrists.

- Arms are fully extended, but elbow remains soft, actually trying to rotate the elbow crease to face toward 12 o'clock.

- Hips align with shoulders, core is engaged and shoulders fall down and away from the ears.

- Abdominals are tight. Think of tipping the tailbone slightly down and away and hollowing out the abdominal wall by drilling the navel to the spine.

- Focus on puffing up the upper back by stretching out the shoulder blades and rounding the shoulders down and out. This will engage the back muscles instead of all the work being done by the shoulders.

©Get Fit Gang, LLC 2020
Katie Wiseman

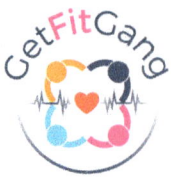

- Tighten the quadriceps and keep core engaged. This will provide a sturdy base.

- Eyes gaze is slightly forward and between the hands.

- Now just breathe and relax into the work! Breath is your fuel. Maintain this still and silent position for the duration of the timed task.

- If you must rest, lift the hips to a downward facing dog, breathe and return to initial position as soon as possible, or you can lower the knees, but return ASAP.

- Continue, focusing on body alignment, arching upper back, shoulders over wrists, breath and a deep contraction of abdominal muscles throughout the timed task.

- Option: Place a ball high between the upper thighs to provide stability to the hips, engage the lower abdominals, inner thighs and to provide a slight inner rotation of the femur bone so knees maintain strict alignment.

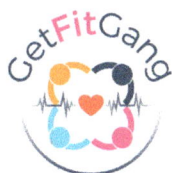

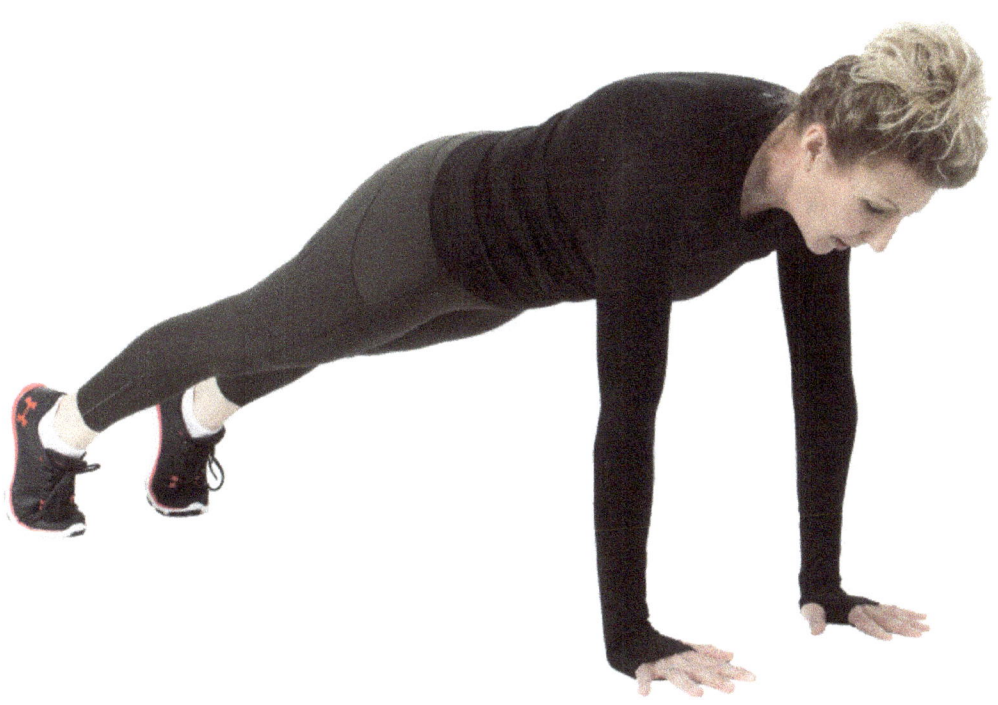

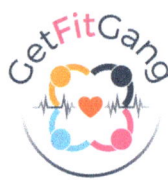

### **Front/Lateral Shoulder Raises: Shoulder girdle**

Front Raises - Complete for the first 45 seconds of the task.
Lateral Raises - Complete for the second 45 seconds of the task.

**Set-Up:**

- Lift lighter set of weights and place them in your hands with palms facing toward upper thighs. Start with 3-5 lbs. As strength increases, weight should also increase.

- Place feet firmly on the ground slightly wider than shoulder width. Knees are actively bent and heels are heavy to provide a solid foundation. Play around with this set-up until you feel really grounded.

- Core is engaged. Visualize a tight core with a slight tilt of the tailbone down and away to flatten the lower back and stabilize the body to control the movement.

- Shoulders are dropped down and away from ears. They do not lift as movement occurs. They must stay down and away, especially as the arms lift the weight.

- The arms are as long as possible, but keep the elbow joint "soft".

- The upper body does not move or sway as weight is lifted. Only the arms move.

**Movement:**

- Initiate movement by contracting the abdominal wall.

- The task begins with front raises. Lift the arms as you raise the weight in front of the body until they are in the same horizontal plane as the shoulder. Visualize tracing an imaginary line with the inside of the weight along the midline of your body.

- Pause briefly at the top of the range of motion and control the weight all the way down to the starting position. Think lift weight to shoulder height, lower to thighs. Exhale at the top of the range of movement and inhale as you control the weight down.

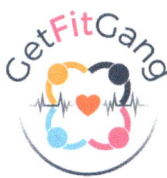

- Repeat this series for 45 seconds.

- At the half way point, move to the lateral muscles of the shoulders. Body alignment is exactly the same, but the weights extend out to the lateral side of the body. Lift weight until arms are in the same horizonal plane as the shoulders, pause and control down.

- Palms face down to the ground or backward to the wall behind you. If you chose to have the palms face backward, you will engage the entire shoulder girdle. Difficult, but worth the extra effort!

- Remember to keep knees bent, core engaged and feet firmly grounded. No swaying!

- You will know you are using the correct weight amount if the last few repetitions are very difficult. Continue, focusing on body alignment, control of the weight, breath and a deep contraction of abdominal muscles throughout the timed task.

- Keep track from one class to the next how many repetitions you are able to accomplish. This will serve as your goal and provide incentive to grow in strength and endurance throughout the year.

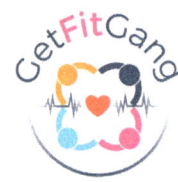

## Front Raises

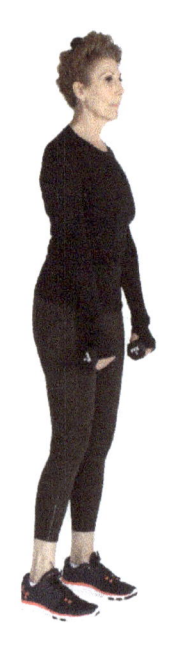
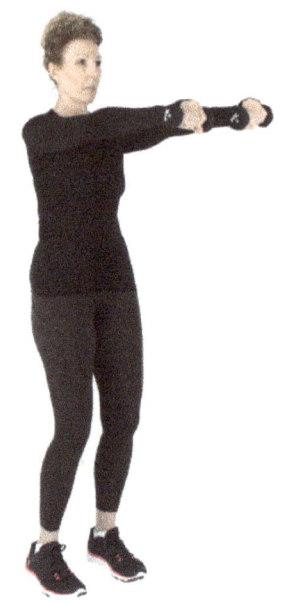

**START**  **END**

## Lateral Raises

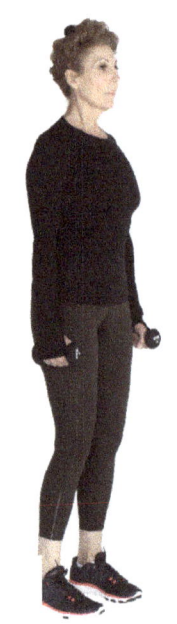
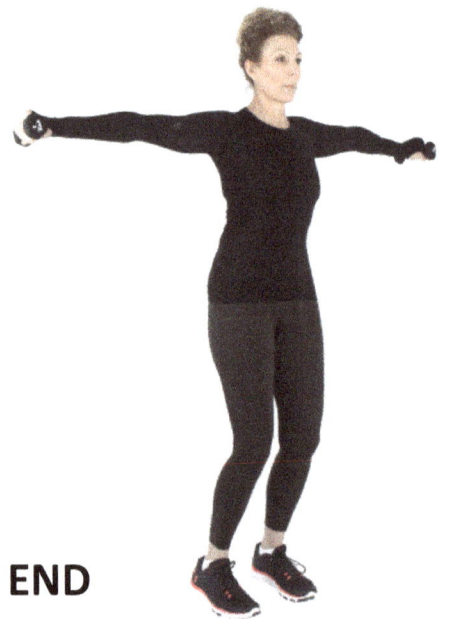

**START**  **END**

Instructional Guide Standard Tasks

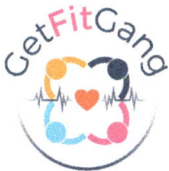

## **Standard Reverse Flys**: Lats and Traps — Upper and Middle Back

Reverse Flys- Complete for the first 45 seconds or throughout entire task.

### Set-Up:

- Lift heavier set of weights, 5 -8 lb., arms extended in front of the body with palms facing each other. Elbows are generously bent.

- Place feet firmly on the ground slightly wider than shoulder width. Knees are actively bent and heels are heavy to provide a solid foundation. Play around with this set-up until you feel really grounded.

- Hinge forward so shoulders fall in front of hips, keeping the chest and heart open and core engaged.

- Keep shoulders dropped down and away from ears.

### Movements:

- Movement is initiated by engaging the core muscles with elbows leading the weight slightly up and back on an arch until the elbows are behind the body and the shoulder blades squeeze together at the top of the range of movement (Visualize holding a pencil between the shoulder blades as the weights are at the top of the range of movement).

- Think of the shape of the arms as if they were hugging a barrel both at the bottom of the movement and at the top of the range of motion. The arms keep this strict form throughout the entire movement.

- Keeping the arms in this barrel shape, lead with the elbows on an arch and focus on squeezing the shoulder blades together at the top, exhale and control the weight back to initial position.

- Exhale at the top of the range of movement and inhale as you control the weights back down to initial position.

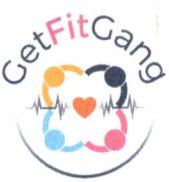

- Upper body remains still, there is no swaying of the body or the weights. Control of the weight occurs with engaged stabilizer muscles (abdominals) while the upper back muscles strengthen.

- Think of tilting the tailbone toward the ground and hollow out the core to elongate the lower back.

- Continue, focusing on body alignment, shoulders down and away from ears, arms in the shape of a barrel, squeezing the shoulder blades at the top of the range of movement, breath and a deep contraction of abdominal muscles throughout the timed task.

- Keep track from one class to the next how many repetitions you are able to accomplish. This will serve as your goal and provide incentive to grow in strength and endurance throughout the year.

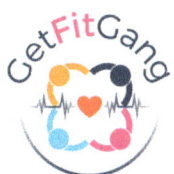

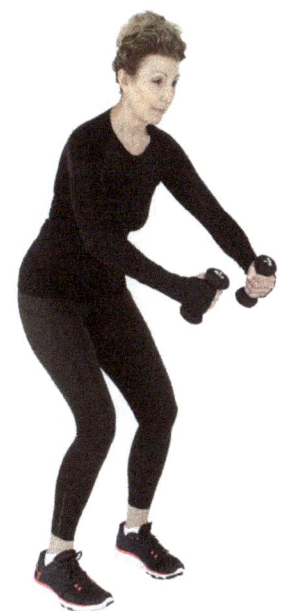

**START**

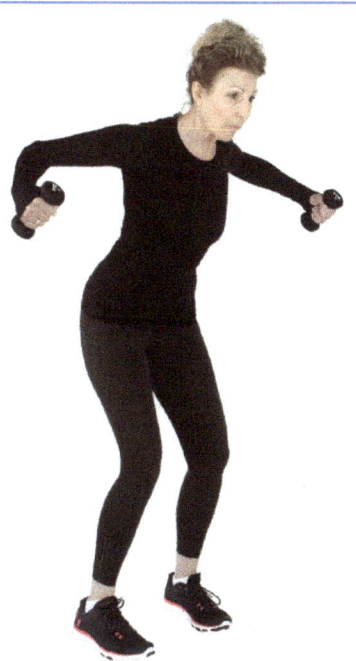

**END**

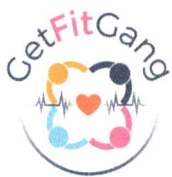

### Scarecrow — Lats and Traps: Upper and middle back

Scarecrow - Complete for the second 45 seconds or throughout entire task.

**Set-Up:**

- Lift heavier set of weights, 5 -8 lb. and place in palms in front of quadriceps, palms facing the quadriceps.

- Place feet firmly on the ground slightly wider than shoulder width. Knees are actively bent and heels are heavy to provide a solid foundation. Play around with this set-up until you feel really grounded.

- Hinge forward so shoulders fall in front of hips, keeping the chest and heart open and core engaged.

- Keep shoulders dropped down and away from ears.

**Movements:**

- Movement is initiated by engaging the core muscles with elbows leading the way up and back. Elbows form a 90-degree angle as weights are lifted and fall directly below or slightly outside the vertical plane of the elbow. The top of the range of motion puts the elbows way behind the body at the same horizontal plane as the shoulder blades, maintaining the strict 90-degree angle at the elbow.

- Shoulder blades squeeze together at the top of the range of movement, exhale and pause. (Visualize holding a pencil between the shoulder blades as the weights are at the top of the range of movement).

- Exhale at the top of the range of movement and inhale as you control the weights back down to initial position, palms facing toward thighs.

- Upper body remains still, there is no swaying of the body or the weights. Control of the body occurs with engaged stabilizer muscles (abdominals), while the upper back muscles strengthen.

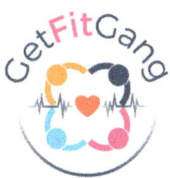

- Continue, focusing on body alignment, shoulders slightly in front of hips, down and away from ears, elbows at a 90-degree angle at the top of the range of movement, shoulder blades squeeze at the top of the range of movement, breath and a deep contraction of abdominal wall throughout the timed task.

- Keep track from one class to the next how many repetitions you are able to accomplish. This will serve as your goal and provide incentive to grow in strength and endurance throughout the year.

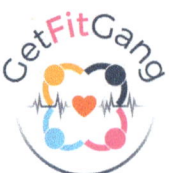

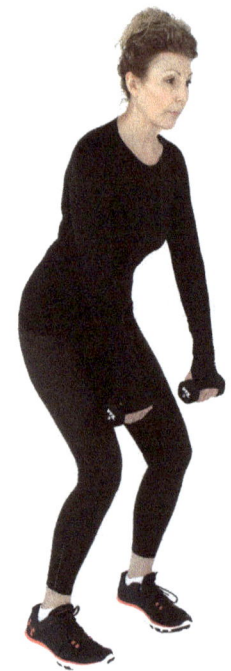

**START**

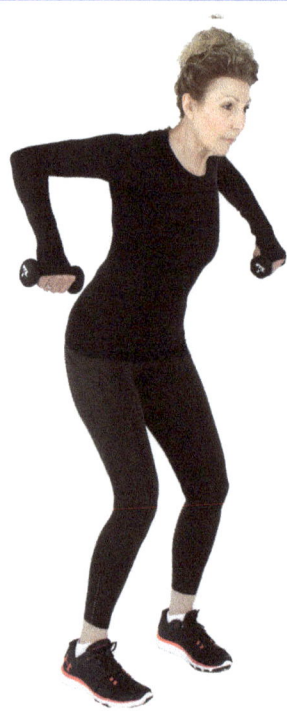

**END**

©Get Fit Gang, LLC 2020
Katie Wiseman

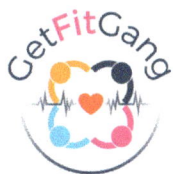

### **Triceps Kickbacks:** Largest muscle of the upper arm

**Set-Up:**

- Lift lighter set of weights, 3-5 lb. and place in palms.

- Lean forward with shoulders in front of hips but keeping heart and chest open. Try not to round shoulders forward, but use back muscles to keep shoulders dropped down and back (think of the pencil between the shoulder blades again). Keep spine straight and heart open.

- Place feet firmly on the ground slightly wider than shoulder width. Knees are actively bent and heels are heavy to provide a solid foundation.

- With weights, bend elbows to a 90 degree angle and lift form behind the body as close as you can to the horizontal plane of the shoulders. Keep heart open, don't lean chest toward ground.

- Wrists stay locked. Don't move them back and forth during the movement. Keep them stable throughout task.

- Visualize reaching elbows up and in toward midline of body.

- Keep shoulders down and away from ears throughout movement.

**Movement:**

- Elbows remain *stationary* as the lower arm extends the weight up and away from the elbow. Elbows are constantly striving to reach up and toward mid-line of body, while shoulders remained dropped down and away from ears.

- Wrists stay locked. Don't move them back and forth during the movement. Keep them stable throughout task.

- Elbows do not move from initial position; only the lower arms extends and retreats. Try not to let the elbows drop during the movement.

©Get Fit Gang, LLC 2020
Katie Wiseman

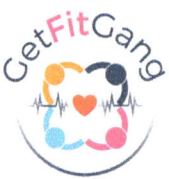

- Squeeze triceps (muscles located at the back of the arm) and pause at the top of the range of movement, with elbow joint fully extended then exhale.

- Inhale as the weight is lowered to the initial position. Control the weight on the way down.

- Don't' swing or sway the upper body or weights. Breath and abdominal muscles should control the weight, not gravity or momentum.

- Continue, focusing on body alignment, shoulders down and away from ears, chest and heart open, elbows high and reaching toward midline, squeeze triceps at the top of the range of motion with elbow joint fully extended, breath and a deep contraction of abdominal muscles throughout the timed task.

- Keep track from one class to the next how many repetitions you are able to accomplish. This will serve as your goal and provide incentive to grow in strength and endurance throughout the year.

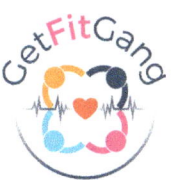

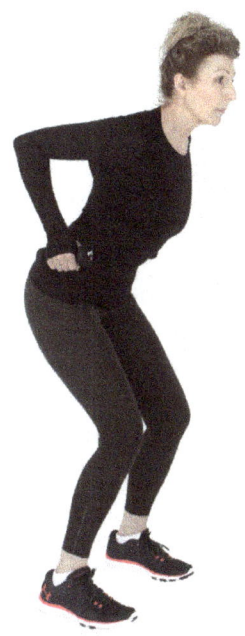

**START**

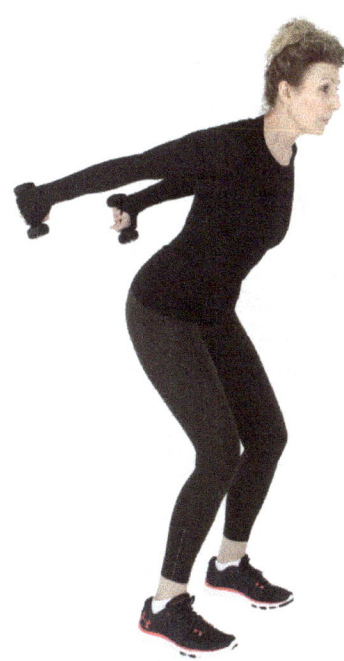

**END**

©Get Fit Gang, LLC 2020
Katie Wiseman

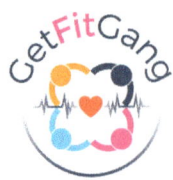

## Lunge: Targets Glutes

**Total Body Strengthener**

### Set – Up:

- Lift heaviest weights available; 8 – 15 lbs. Place in hands.
- Place the body where you have enough room to take a large step forward.
- Shoulders are stacked over hips, hips over knees, knees over ankles.
- Engage core, chest and heart open and shoulders down and away from ears.

### Movement:
- Keep arms extended with weights to the sides of the body.
- Take a large (over extended) step forward, keeping shoulders stacked on top of hips.
- Lower the hips by dropping the *back* knee toward the ground, until the front thigh is parallel to the floor.
- Make sure the front knee does not slide forward beyond the front shoe laces. Ideally, you want to keep the knee stacked directly over the front ankle. If you have to widen your stance by sliding the back foot backward before you lower the legs to ensure proper knee alignment for the front knee, that is fine.
- After you reach your desired depth, contract the abdominals as you exhale, *driving* the front heel into the ground, keeping arms extended at sides and return to a standing position.
- Step forward with the other foot and repeat.

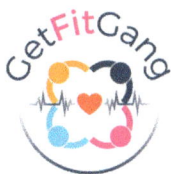

- Keep shoulders stacked over hips as best as you can throughout the movement. The shoulders can sneak forward a little as you return to initial position, but not much. We want to prevent stress on the lower back.

- This exercise can challenge the knee joint. Only go deep enough to maintain strong body alignment. If you find any discomfort in the knee joint, discontinue the standard lunge and try either Phase 1 or Phase 2 of the modified lunge instead.

- During the 90 second series, aim to complete 16-20 repetitions, stepping forward with one foot, then the other. In a small space, take a step forward, complete the lunge, then simply turn the body back around and repeat.

- Continue, focusing on body alignment, shoulders down and away from ears, chest and heart open, front thigh parallel to the floor, front knee over front ankle, exhale on the way up, inhale on the way down and a deep contraction of abdominal muscles throughout the timed task.

- Keep track from one class to the next how many repetitions you are able to accomplish. This will serve as your goal and provide incentive to grow in strength and endurance throughout the year.

©Get Fit Gang, LLC 2020
Katie Wiseman

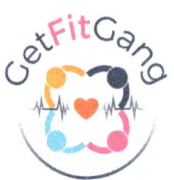

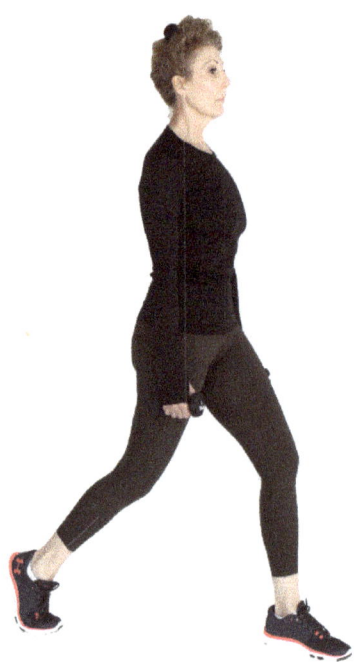

**START**

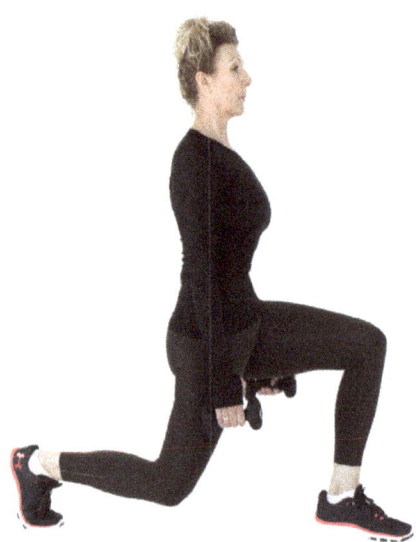

**END**

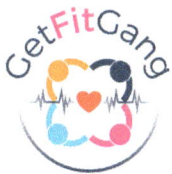

## **Squats:** Performed with or without weights — Thighs and Glutes

**Total Body Strengthener**

**Set – Up:**

- Choose heaviest weight you can manage; 8 – 15 lbs. Place in hands.

- Feet are wider than shoulder width apart, heels deeply grounded. If you can't keep heels grounded due to flexibility of the ankle joint, place a large 2" rectangular block, some books (make sure they are the same size book) or flat bar weights under each heel to ensure adequate pressure can be placed on each heel during movement.

- In a wide, but comfortable stance, feet face toward 11 o'clock and 1 o'clock. During movement, knees track in the same line as the feet, with the knee facing toward the middle toes at the depth of movement.

- Engage core, keeping chest and heart open and shoulders down and away from ears.

**Movement:**

- Initiate movement by engaging the core and push hips way *back* and away from feet.

- As the hips extend back and away from the feet, lift the weight to mid-chest to provide counter balance to the position. If you aren't using weights, lift the arms.

- Lower the hips until the thighs are parallel to the ground, however, do not allow the knees to move in front of the laces of your shoes or by transferring weight into the toes. Keep grounded in the heels, with core deeply engaged.

- The ideal is for the thighs to be parallel to the floor, however, only go deep enough to feel stable and safe.

- The shoulders will fall in front of the hips as the core stabilizes the movement and the weights are lifted to the alignment of mid-chest, but still try to keep heart open.

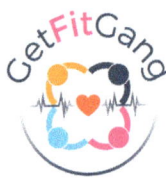

- To return to starting position, exhale forcefully and drive the heels into the ground (or object) as you extend the legs and bring the hips up, then tilt them slightly forward (keep core deeply engaged here to protect the lower back) for deep glute engagement.

- Once you have reached the top of the range of motion, the legs fully extend, but the knees remain soft.

- At the top of the range of movement, tilt the tailbone toward the ground and squeeze the glutes. This slight "tip" will deeply engage the abdominals and flatten out the lower back.

- Take a deep cleansing breathe at the top and repeat.

- Establish a consistent pace. Try not to rest too long at the completion of the movement. Your body craves oxygen during this type of muscular intensity; breathe deeply during this full body task to develop deep strength in all the major muscle groups of the body.

- Continue, focusing on body alignment, breath and a deep contraction of abdominal muscles throughout the timed task.

- Keep track from one class to the next how many repetitions you are able to accomplish. This will serve as your goal and provide incentive to grow in strength and endurance throughout the year.

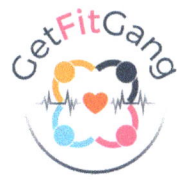

## Squats With Weights

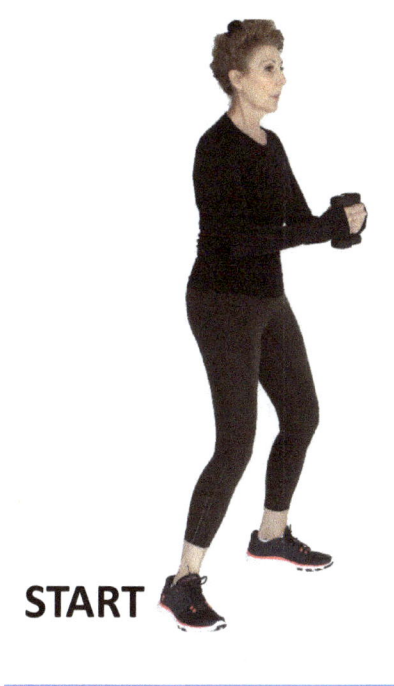
**START**

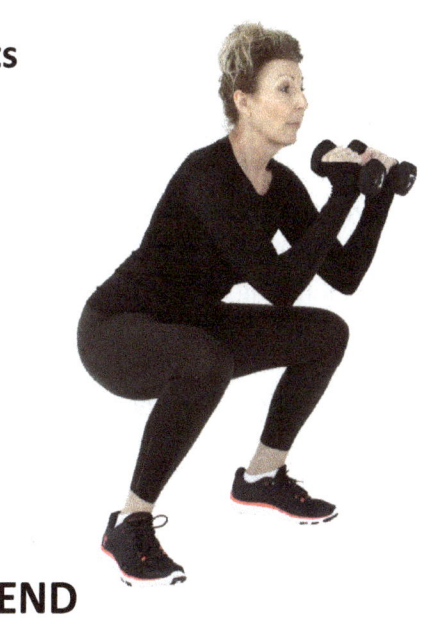
**END**

## Squats Without Weights

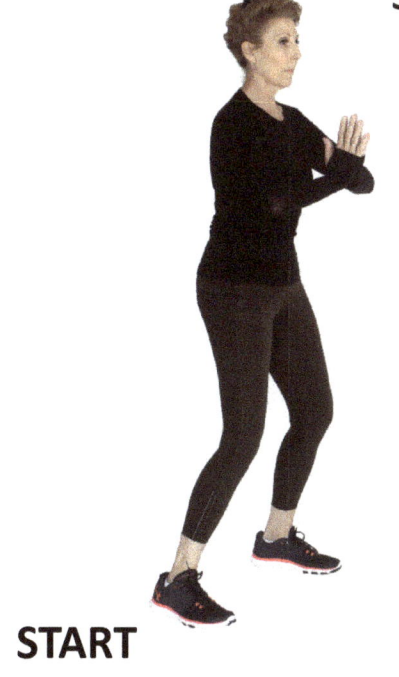
**START**

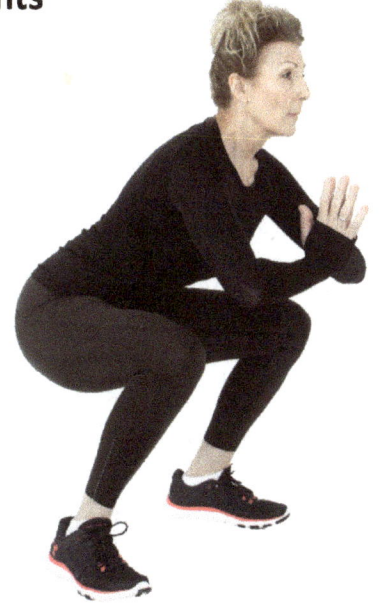
**END**

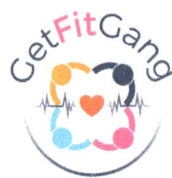

### Step Series: Increases Cardiovascular Strength and Endurance

The step phase of the Get Fit Gang fitness program is designed to elevate the heart rate. Strive to work as hard as you can to get the blood pumping throughout the body. Maintain a rhythm of movement for the entirety of the cycle. Focus on the music to help with engagement and rhythm. Remember, increasing the heart rate is the name of the game here! Taking this elevated heart rate to the strength training tasks will enhance the entire program.

There are several ways in which to perform the step series. I will outline each type below:

### Standard Step Up

Use this form if you desire to keep this portion of the workout low impact. You can easily elevate the heart rate without jumping or stepping rapidly. All you need to do to ensure a heightened heart rate is to keep your arms above your heart. Keep shoulders dropped down and back and heart remains open, but arms stay up above the heart throughout the 90 second task. I promise this will elevate the heart rate and keep little impact on the knee joints.

- Step up with one foot, leaning shoulders ever so slightly in front of hips, but heart remains open, core engaged.
- Place entire foot on step.
- Exhale as you step up, inhale as you return to starting position and alternate feet.
- Make sure you switch lead feet after each series. If you start with the right in series one, start with the left in series two.
- Place arms in the shape of a goal post and lift elbows until they are in alignment, or slightly above the heart.

### Step Jumps (Photo example included)

This is one of my preferred methods to use during the step series of the program. It engages the thighs, glutes and abdominals and elevates the heart effectively.

- Place ball and arch of the foot onto the step with heel slightly off the step.

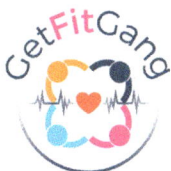

- Upper body will be slightly in front of the hips, with the core tightly engaged.
- Explode from the front foot on the step, going straight up into the air and switch legs mid-air as you return to starting position (much easier to do than it sounds).
- Exhale as you explode up and inhale as you come back to starting position.

## Box Jumps

The youngsters seem to love this! Think of plyometrics (box jumping) and you'll get the picture. This requires a large amount of explosive power and will deeply engage the thighs, glutes, abdominals and most importantly, heart rate. Try it, you may love it!

- Stand directly in front of steps, with hips, knees, shoulders and feet squared to steps.
- Feet are slightly wider than shoulder width, knees are strongly bent, and core engaged.
- Inhale deeply, lower the hips (think small squat) and explode up toward steps, exhaling as you land with both feet squarely in the middle of the steps.
- Step down carefully and repeat.

## Side Jumps

This is my other most favorite type of step series to use. It deeply engages the glutes (largest muscles of the body…so the heart rate is quickly elevated). The movement can be slow and controlled and you do not have to complete as many repetitions as with the other steps' series explained above. The key to this series is to stay low the entire time.

- Hips are squared to the small edge of the step.
- Place one foot on the step and lower the hips to a squat position. Arms are extended out and toward the front of the body.
- Explode off the foot on the step and slide the hips laterally toward the opposite side of the step as you switch feet (again, it's much easier to perform than it sounds).
- Stay low and in a squat position as you alternate from foot to foot, moving laterally.
- Exhale as you move; inhale in the squat phase on each side of the step and repeat.

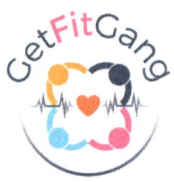

## Step Jumps

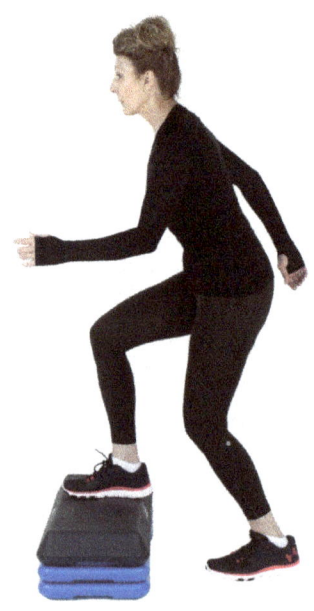

**START**

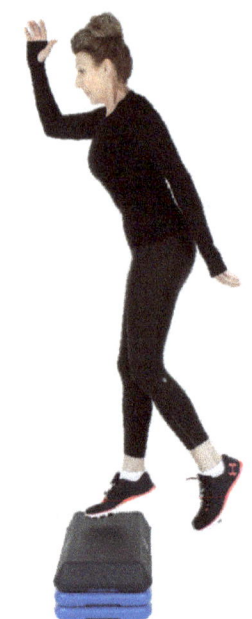

**END**

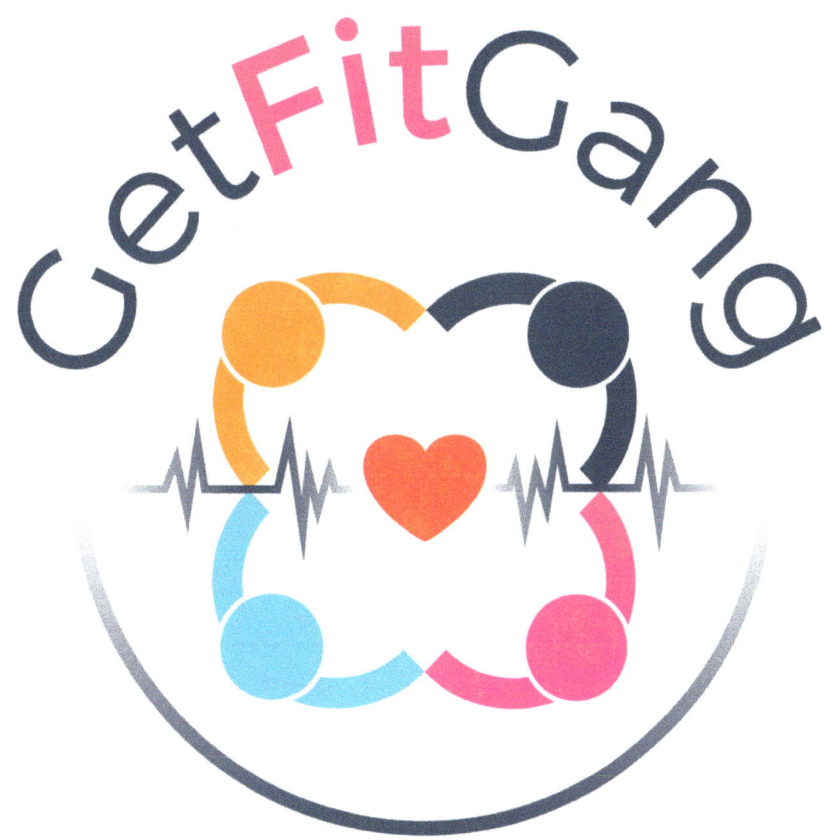

# Instructional Guide
# Modified Tasks

©Get Fit Gang, LLC 2020
Katie Wiseman

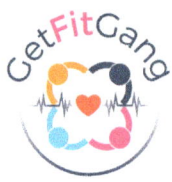

# Instructional Guide – Modified Tasks

Instructional Guide – Demonstration and application of techniques and skills.

**Modified Tasks** ............................................................................................. 70

    **Push Up** ............................................................................................. 71
        I. Push Up at Wall ............................................................................ 71

    **Abdominals** ....................................................................................... 74
        I. Curl ................................................................................................ 74
        II. Scissor Legs .................................................................................. 77

    **Forearm Plank** .................................................................................. 80

    **Bridge Without Band** ...................................................................... 82

    **Straight Arm Plank** .......................................................................... 84

    **Shoulder Raises** ............................................................................... 87
        I. Front Raises .................................................................................. 87
        II. Lateral Raises .............................................................................. 87

    **Upper-Mid Back** ............................................................................... 90
        I. Reverse Fly .................................................................................... 90
        II. Scarecrow .................................................................................... 93

    **Triceps Kickback** .............................................................................. 96

    **Lunges at Steps** ............................................................................... 99

    **Squats at Wall w/Ball** ..................................................................... 102

©Get Fit Gang, LLC 2020
Katie Wiseman

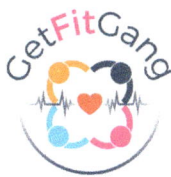

## Modified Push Ups at wall: Total Body Strengthener

**Set-Up:**

- Place hands on the wall, wider than shoulder width, but within the same horizonal plane as the shoulders.

- Place entire hand onto the wall opening the fingers by extending the webbing between the fingers and placing all knuckles on the wall, especially the index and thumb to help protect the wrists.

- Move hips and feet back from the wall as far as possible while still keeping hands in contact with the wall.

- Come up as high as possible onto the toes, keeping knees soft and knee caps facing toward wall.

- Abdominals are tight. Think of tipping the tailbone slightly down and away and hollowing out the abdominal wall by drilling the navel to the spine.

- Eyes gaze is slightly above the fingers on a mid-point of the wall.

**Movement:**

- Think of the movement as a moving plank…the entire body "form" moves down and up, not just chest, or chin.

- Lead with the sternum (chest) by bending the elbows, keeping core engaged and lower as far as possible without collapsing either the abdominals or shoulders    (Note: only go as deep as strict form will allow…as strength is gained, depth will increase).

- Extend arms fully at the top of the movement, but elbows remain soft.

- Inhale as the body moves down and exhale forcefully as the body returns…fill up and release each time….breathing is fuel for your body during movement; this will ensure your body can stay engaged throughout the 90 second interval.

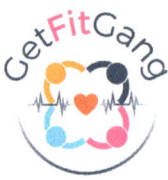

- Stay high up on toes to engage thighs.

- If possible, catch the beat of the music and move with the rhythm.

- Move as controlled as possible…don't rush through the movement. Slow and steady gets the job done.

- Continue, focusing on body alignment, breath and a deep contraction of abdominal muscles throughout the timed task.

- Keep track from one class to the next how many repetitions you are able to accomplish. This will serve as your goal and provide incentive to grow in strength and endurance throughout the year.

- Option: Place a ball high between the upper thighs to provide stability to the hips, engage the lower abdominals, inner thighs and to provide a slight inner rotation of the femur bone so knees maintain strict alignment.

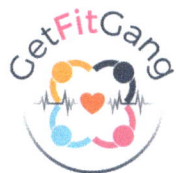

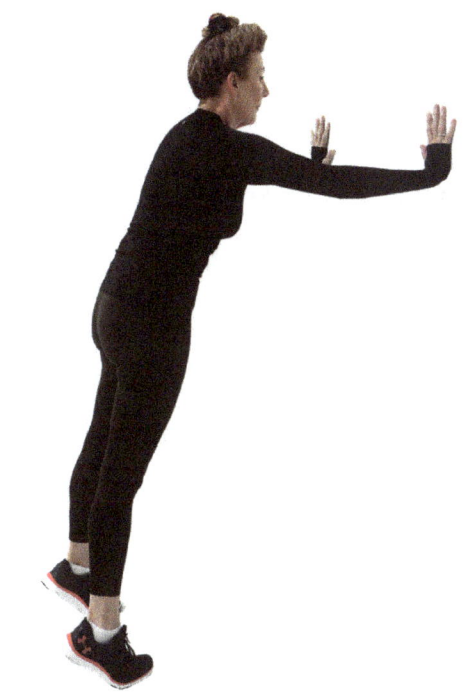

**START**

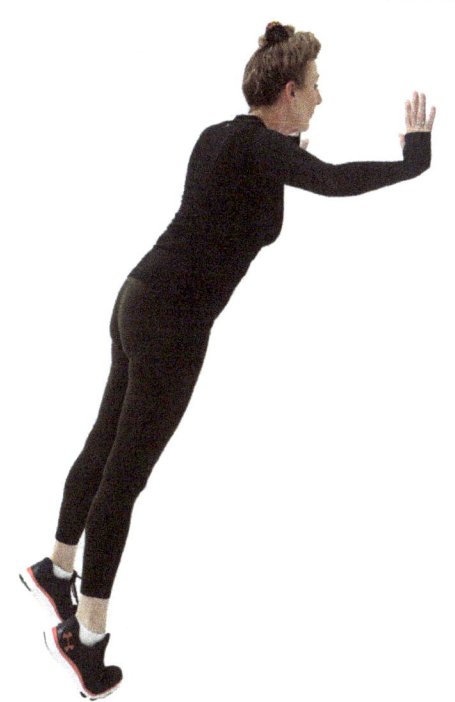

**END**

©Get Fit Gang, LLC 2020
Katie Wiseman

Instructional Guide Modified Tasks

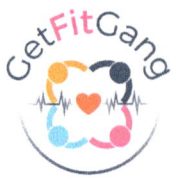

## Modified Abdominal Curl

### Set-Up:

- Lay down on mat, facing up with knees bent to allow sacrum (flat bone at the base of the spine) to be in contact with the mat.

- Place hands to the sides of your body, palms down.

- Visualize an apple between your chin and chest. Try to prevent dropping your chin toward your chest, so the work stays in abdominals, not the neck.

### Movement:

- Visualize drilling the navel to the spine to initiate the movement, then lift the shoulder blades as high off the mat as possible, reaching the chest (sternum) toward the ceiling, maintaining tight upper abdominals, all without dropping the chin toward the chest.

- Slide the hands toward the heels by lifting the shoulder blades off the mat and focus on pushing the abdominal wall down into the mat. Don't just reach the arms forward, the arms follow the lifting of the shoulders.

- Exhale as you lift the shoulders and inhale as you return to the mat.

- Rest your head on the mat between repetitions to give the neck muscles a rest.

- Breathing pattern is paramount to keep abdominals contracting in the correct sequence.

- Pause briefly at the top of the range of movement as you exhale by drilling the navel to the spine and pushing the lower back even further into the mat.

- Make a mental connection between your body and mind throughout the movement. This focus will help deepen the muscular engagement and help regulate your breath.

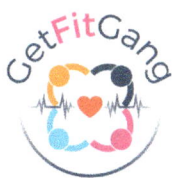

- Range of movement is not large, you are just lifting the shoulder blades off the mat, reaching the chest toward the ceiling. A burning sensation will be felt in the upper abdominals fairly quickly when movement and breathe coordinate.

- Try not to rush through the movement and focus on your breath. Quality of movement, especially with mental focus, wins over quantity.

- Continue, focusing on body alignment, breath and a deep contraction of abdominal muscles throughout the timed task.

- Keep track from one class to the next how many repetitions you are able to accomplish. This will serve as your goal and provide incentive to grow in strength and endurance throughout the year.

- Option: Place a ball high between the upper thighs to provide stability to the hips, engage the lower abdominals, inner thighs and to provide a slight inner rotation of the femur bone so knees maintain strict alignment.

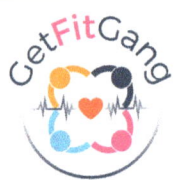

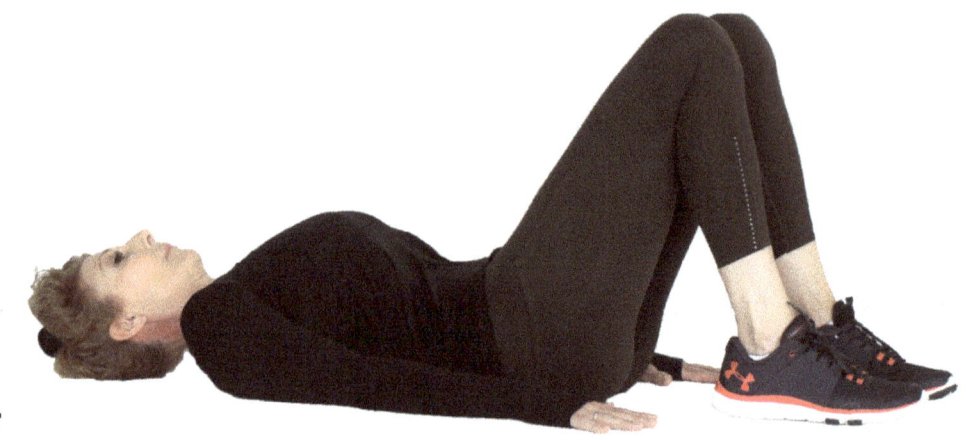

**START**

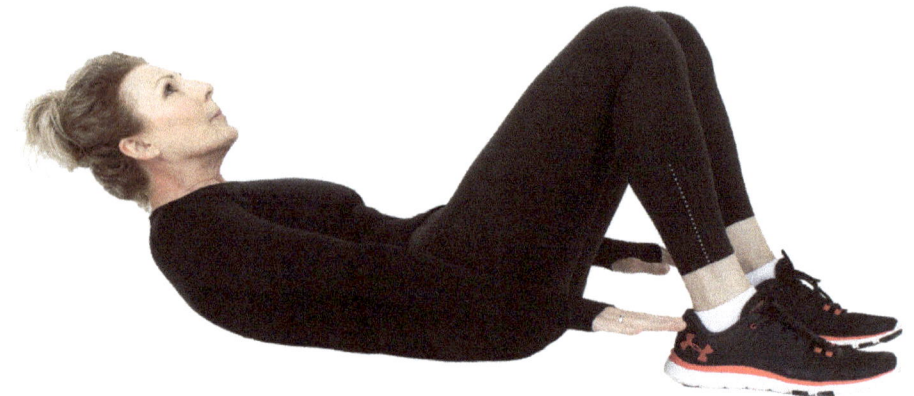

**END**

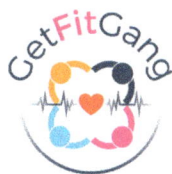

## Modified Abdominals Scissor Legs

Complete for the second 45 seconds of the task.

**Set-Up:**

- Lay down on back and extend legs into the air directly above the hips.
- Place hands under sacrum (flat bone located at the base of the spine) for support.
- Rest head on mat.
- Engage abdominals by tilting hip bones toward shoulders, elongating the lower back and hollowing out core.
- Slight bend in the knee to keep movement in the lower abdominals and out of the hip flexors.
- Point toes toward ceiling.

**Movement:**

- Initiate movement by engaging abdominals and visualize drilling the navel to the spine. This slight movement will flatten the lower back out even more and engage the deep transverse abdominals.
- Lower one leg at a time as far as possible without touching the ground or allowing the lower back to arch or rise off the mat.
- Exhale at the bottom of the range of movement and re-engage the abdominals to raise the leg back to the starting position.

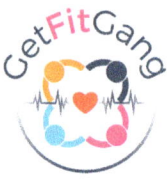

- Repeat series using the other leg.

- Raise the head, neck and shoulders, if possible, to deepen engagement of abdominal wall.

- Focus on rhythmic breathing throughout the movement.

- Control of movement is important…don't just let the leg drop allowing gravity to do the work. Use the core muscles to control the full range of movement, throughout.

- Continue, focusing on body alignment, breath and a deep contraction of abdominal muscles throughout the timed task.

- Keep track from one class to the next how many repetitions you are able to accomplish. This will serve as your goal and provide incentive to grow in strength and endurance throughout the year.

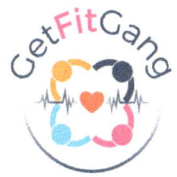

**START**

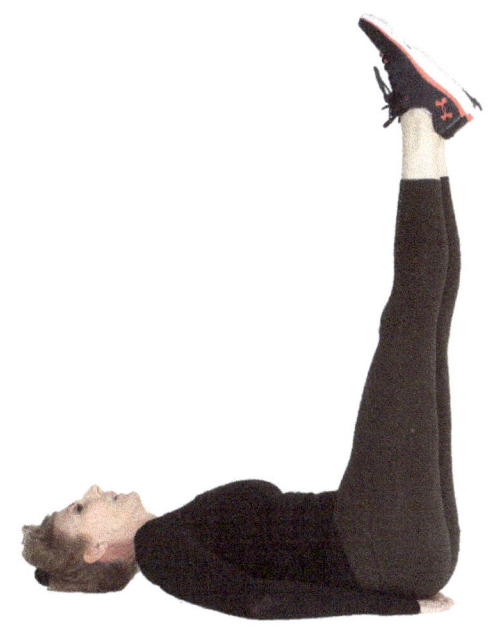

**END**

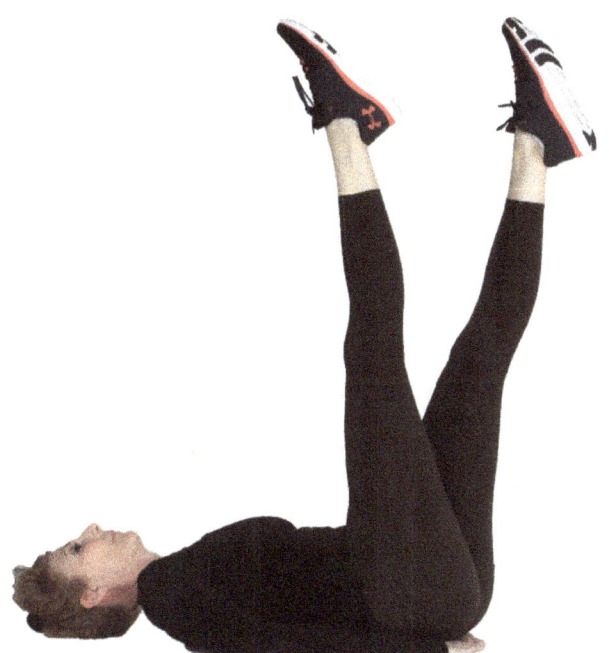

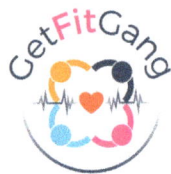

## **Modified Forearm Plank:** Total Body Strengthener

**Set-Up:** There is no movement with this task.

- Place elbows on mat creating the number eleven (train tracks) with elbows slightly inside the vertical plane of the shoulders.
- Place your knees on the mat and engage the abdominals (Phase 1). Your abdominals serve as a "wall" to support your spine. Abdominal engagement is key to the exercise.
- Place entire forearm and entire hand, including finger pads and joints firmly on the mat.
- Lift the hips, but keep knees on the mat and stack shoulders over elbows.
- Abdominals are tight. Think of tipping the tailbone slightly down and away by hollowing out the core by drilling navel to spine.
- Focus on puffing up the upper back by rounding out the shoulder blades and dropping the shoulders. This will allow recruitment of back muscles.
- Eyes gaze is slightly up and between the hands.
- Breath is your fuel. Maintain this still and silent position for the duration of the 90 seconds.
- If you can lift the knees, even for a brief time (Phase 2), do that by extending the legs behind you, drop your toes and lift the knees slightly off the mat and hold. This will escalate the strengthening process so you can quickly gain enough strength to complete the standard forearm plank.
- For me, this is the most difficult task in the entire series. This is an isometric contraction of the muscular system (working muscles without movement) and a highly effective strength builder.
- Continue, focusing on body alignment, arching upper back, shoulders stacked over wrists, breath and a deep contraction of abdominal muscles throughout the timed task.
- Option: Place a ball high between the upper thighs to provide stability to the hips, engage the lower abdominals, inner thighs and to provide a slight inner rotation of the femur bone so knees maintain strict alignment.

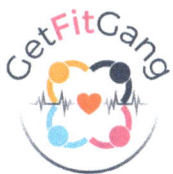

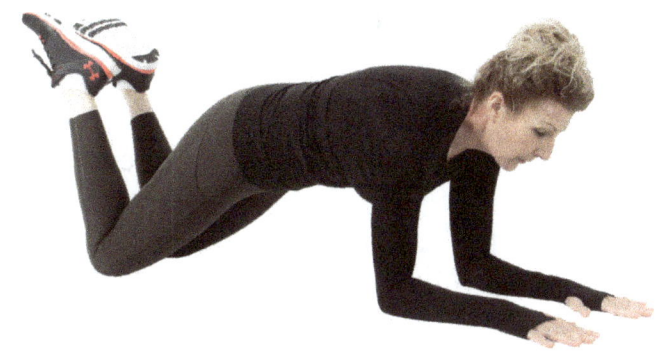

PHASE 1

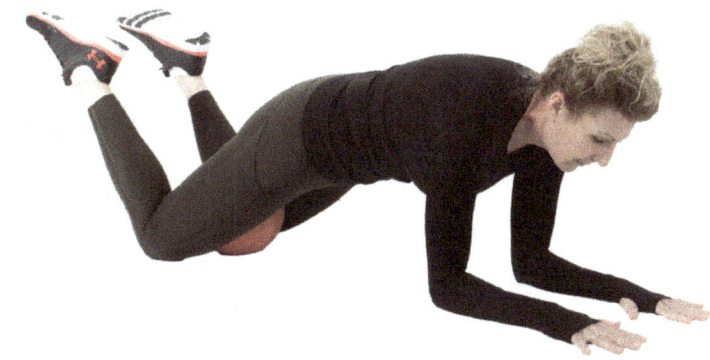

PHASE 1
WITH BALL

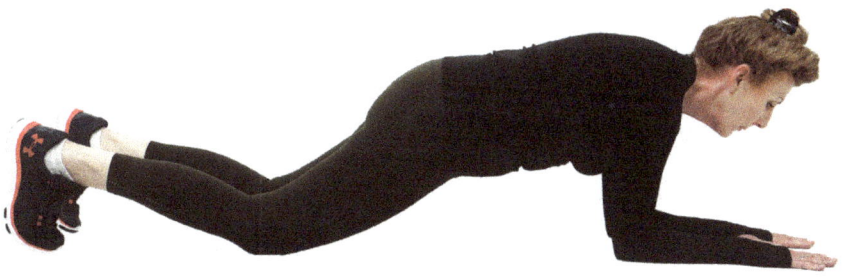

PHASE 2
LIFT KNEES
BRIEFLY

Instructional Guide Modified Tasks

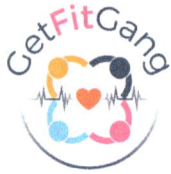

## **Modified Bridge without Band:** Glute Maximus and Medius

**Set-Up:**

- Lay down on your back, resting your head on the mat with arms resting at sides of the body.
- Bend your knees, place ball between upper thighs and place your feet hip width apart off the mat and onto the floor.

**Movement:**

- Movement is initiated when you engage abdominal wall by drilling navel to spine, elongating the back against the mat.
- Dig your heels into the floor as you squeeze the ball and lift your hips, keeping knees in alignment with hip joint.
- With core tightly engaged, lift the hips as high as you can while keeping mid back and shoulders on the mat and maintaining the small tilt of the hip bones toward shoulders.
- The movement continues as the hips come up, while the mid and upper back maintain contact on mat, then return to initial position.
- Squeezing the ball will allow the knees, hips and shoulders to be in a straight vertical line at the top of the range of movement. This line will become "cleaner" as strength is developed.
- Consciously squeeze the glutes *and* the ball at the top of the range of motion.
- Exhale at the top of the movement and inhale as the hips make their way back down to the mat.
- Continue, focusing on body alignment, breath and contraction of the glute muscles throughout the timed task.
- Keep track from one class to the next how many repetitions you are able to accomplish. This will serve as your goal and provide incentive to grow in strength and endurance throughout the year.

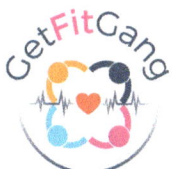

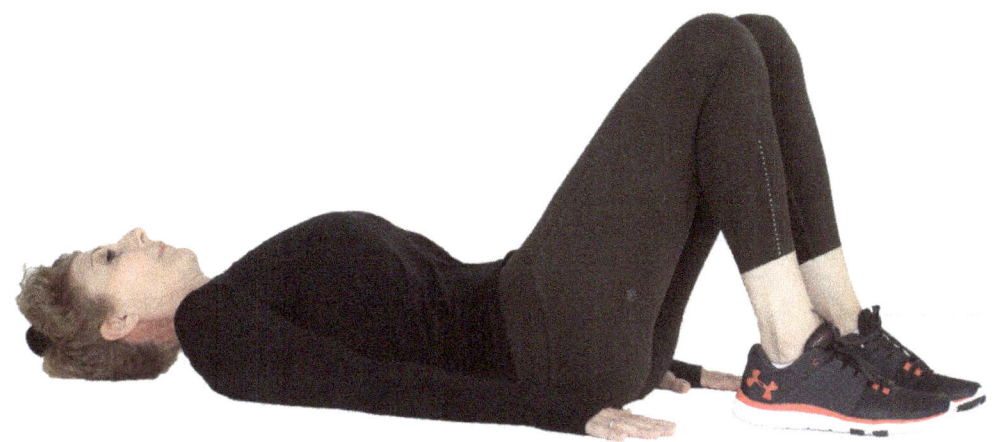

**START**

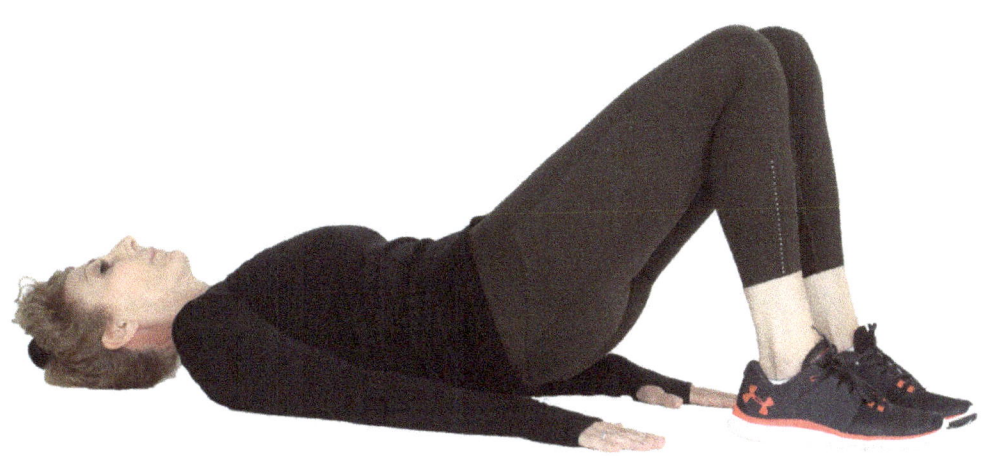

**END**

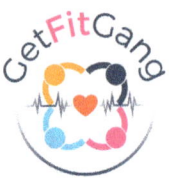

### **Straight Arm Plank:** Total Body Strengthener

**Set-Up:** There is no movement with this task.

- This task will be done using a mat on the floor.

- Place hands on floor off the mat.

- Place entire hand, including finger pads and joints firmly on the floor. Be sure to expand the webbing of the hand and press squarely into the floor with both hands equally.

- Bend knees, placing meaty part of thigh above the knee joint onto the mat with knees hip width distance apart by moving the shoulders directly above the wrists (Phase 1).

- Contract your abdominals and quadriceps as you think of drilling your navel to your spine to hollow out your core and expand your shoulder blades out as you drop your shoulders down.

- Your abdominals serve as a "wall" to support your spine. With your knees on the mat, more focus most be on a hard contraction of the core. Think of hollowing out and rounding the back, focusing on tilting hips toward shoulders and drilling navel to spine.

- Do not allow the shoulders to fall behind the wrists, but keep soft bend in the elbow.

- Core remains engaged and shoulders fall down and away from the ears.

- Focus on puffing up the upper back by stretching out the shoulder blades and rounding the shoulders. This will engage the large muscles of the back.

- Tighten the quadriceps and keep core engaged. This will provide a study base.

- Eyes gaze is slightly forward and between the hands.

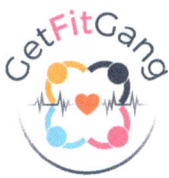

- If you can lift the knees, even for a brief time (Phase 2), do that by extending the legs behind you, drop your toes and lift the knees slightly off the mat and hold. This will escalate the strengthening process so you can quickly gain enough strength to complete the standard straight arm plank.

- Now just breathe. Breath is your fuel. Maintain this still and silent position for the duration of the timed task.

- If you must rest, slide hips down to a child's pose, resting hips on heels, breathe and return to initial position as soon as possible.

- Continue, focusing on body alignment, arching upper back, shoulders over wrists, breath and a deep contraction of abdominal muscles throughout the timed task.

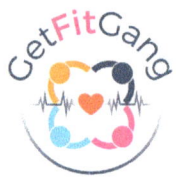

*Instructional Guide Modified Tasks*

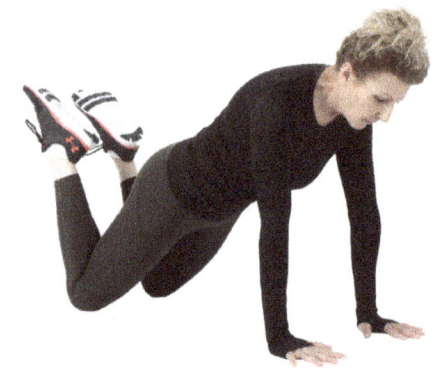

PHASE 1

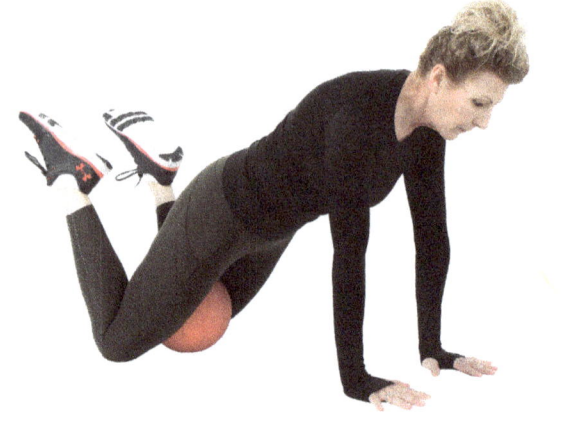

PHASE 1
WITH BALL

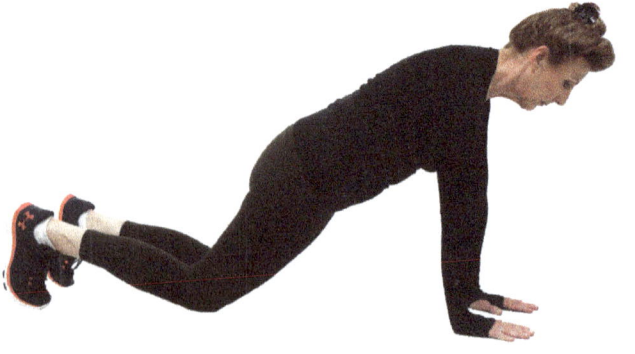

PHASE 2
LIFTING KNEES
BRIEFLY

©Get Fit Gang, LLC 2020
Katie Wiseman

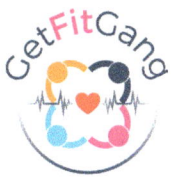

## **Modified Front/Lateral Shoulder Raises:** Shoulder Girdle

Front Raises — Complete for the first 45 seconds of the task.

Lateral Raises — Complete for the second 45 seconds of the task.

**Set-Up:**

- No weights will be used. We will use body weight to strengthen the shoulder girdle until adequate strength is gained.

- Place feet firmly on the ground slightly wider than shoulder width. Knees are actively bent and heels are heavy to provide a solid foundation. Play around with this set-up until you feel really grounded.

- Core is engaged. Visualize a tight core with a slight tilt of the tailbone down and away to flatten the lower back and stabilize the body to control the movement.

- Shoulders are dropped down and away from ears. They do not lift as movement occurs. They must stay down and away, especially as the arms lift.

- The arms are as long as possible, but keep the elbow joint "soft".

- The upper body does not move or sway as weight is lifted. Only the arms move.

**Movement:**

- Initiate movement by contracting the abdominals.

- The task begins with front raises. Raise your arms in front of the body until they are in the same horizonal plane as the shoulder.

- Pause at the top of the range of motion, with shoulder down and away and arms fully extended, slowly and methodically twist the palms up and down keeping arms straight with a soft bend in the elbow.

©Get Fit Gang, LLC 2020
Katie Wiseman

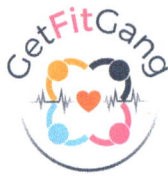

- Focus on your breath, keeping shoulders down and away from ears and abdominals tightly engaged. Tight abdominals will be the key to completing this exercise.

- Repeat twisting your palms up and down for 45 seconds. Drop arms only if necessary, and begin again as soon as your shake your arms and shoulders out.

- After a brief rest, extend arms to the sides of the body (lateral raises) and repeat the twisting movement for the remaining 45 seconds.

- Keep track from one class to the next how long you are able to accomplish holding your arms up. When you can sustain the movement for the full 45 seconds, it's time to add weights!

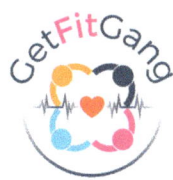

## Frontal Shoulder Raises

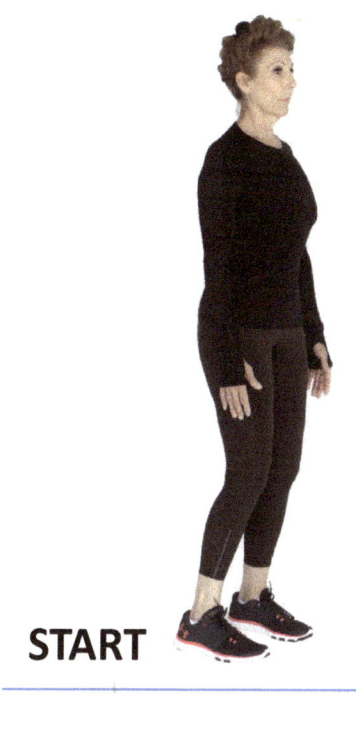
**START**

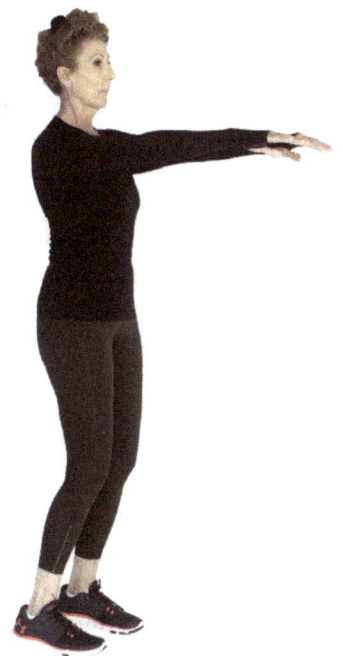
**END**

## Lateral Shoulder Raises

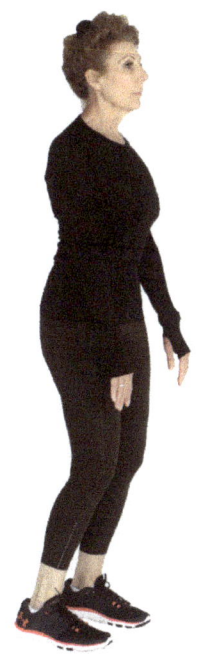
**START**

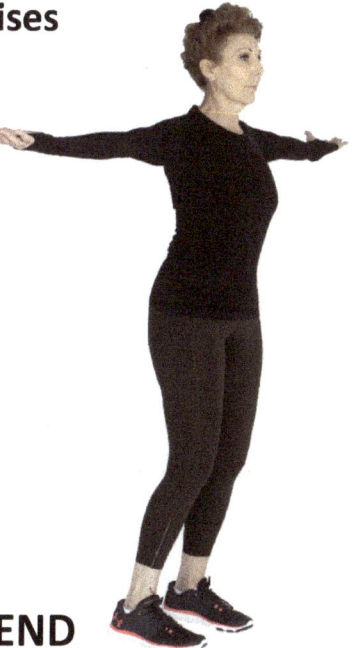
**END**

*Instructional Guide Modified Tasks*

©Get Fit Gang, LLC 2020
Katie Wiseman

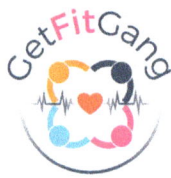

## **Modified Reverse Flys**: Lats and Traps — Upper and Middle Back

Reverse Flys- Complete for the first 45 seconds or throughout entire task.

### Set-Up:

- Lift lighter set of weights, 2-4 lb., or you may choose to do this task without weights. Extend arms in front of the thighs, palms facing each other. Elbows are generously bent.

- Place feet firmly on the ground slightly wider than shoulder width. Knees are actively bent, and heels are heavy to provide a solid foundation. Play around with this set-up until you feel really grounded.

- Hinge forward so shoulders fall slightly in front of hips, but keep the chest and heart open and core engaged.

- Keep shoulders dropped down and away from ears.

### Movements:

- Movement is initiated by engaging the core muscles with elbows leading the way slightly up and back on an arch until the elbows are behind the body and the shoulder blades squeeze together at the top of the range of movement (Visualize holding a pencil between the shoulder blades at the top of the range of motion).

- Think of the shape of the arms as if they were hugging a barrel both at the bottom of the movement and at the top of the range of motion. The arms keep this strict form throughout the entire movement.

- Exhale at the top of the range of movement and inhale as you control the weights back down to initial position, palms facing toward thighs.

- Upper body remains still, there is no swinging of the body or the weights. Control of the body occurs with stabilizer muscles (abdominals) while the upper back muscles and breath control the weight.

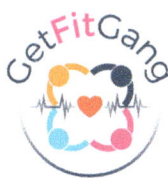

- Continue, focusing on body alignment, shoulders down and away from ears, arms in the shape of a barrel, squeezing the shoulder blades at the top of the range of movement with breath and a deep contraction of abdominal muscles a focus throughout the timed task.

- Keep track from one class to the next how many repetitions you are able to accomplish. This will serve as your goal and provide incentive to grow in strength and endurance throughout the year.

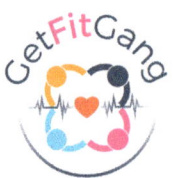

Instructional Guide Modified Tasks

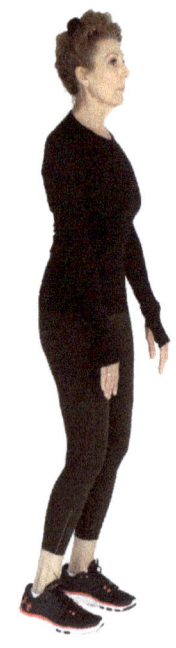

**START**

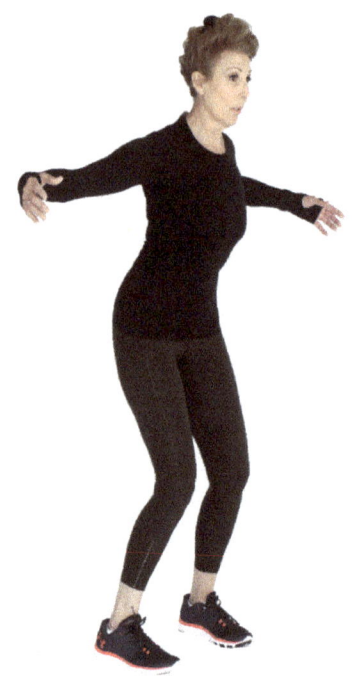

**END**

©Get Fit Gang, LLC 2020
Katie Wiseman

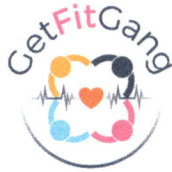

## Modified Scarecrow — Lats and Traps — Upper and middle back

Scarecrow — Complete for the second 45 seconds or throughout entire task.

### Set-Up:

- Lift lighter set of weights, 2-4 lb., or you may choose to do this task without weights. Extend arms in front of the thighs, palms facing each other. Elbows are generously bent.

- Place feet firmly on the ground wider than shoulder width. Knees are actively bent and heels are heavy to provide a solid foundation. Play around with this set-up until you feel really grounded.

- Hinge forward so shoulders fall slightly in front of hips, keeping the chest and heart open and core engaged.

- Keep shoulders dropped down and away from ears.

### Movements:

- Movement is initiated by engaging the core muscles, elbows leading the way up and back. Elbows form a 90 degree angle as weights fall directly below or slightly outside the plane of the elbow. The top of the range of motion puts the elbows way behind the body at the same horizontal plane as the shoulders blades, maintaining the strict 90 degree angle at the elbow.

- Shoulder blades squeeze together at the top of the range of movement, pause and exhale (Visualize holding a pencil between the shoulder blades at the top of the range of motion).

- Exhale at the top of the range of movement and inhale as you control the weight back down to initial position, palms facing toward thighs.

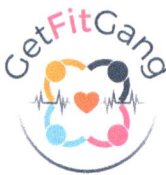

- Upper body remains still, there is no swinging of the body or the weights. Control of the body occurs with stabilizer muscles (abdominals) while the upper back muscles and breath control the weights.

- Continue, focusing on body alignment, shoulders down and away from ears, elbows at a 90 degree angle at the top of the range of movement, breath and a deep contraction of abdominal muscles throughout the timed task.

- Keep track from one class to the next how many repetitions you are able to accomplish. This will serve as your goal and provide incentive to grow in strength and endurance throughout the year.

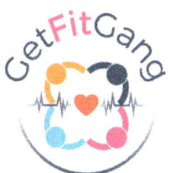

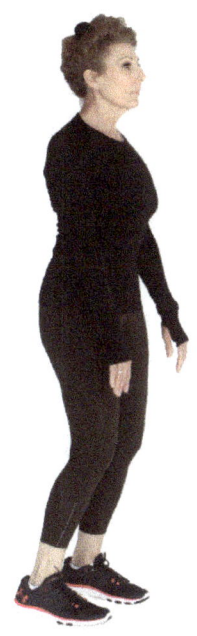

**START**

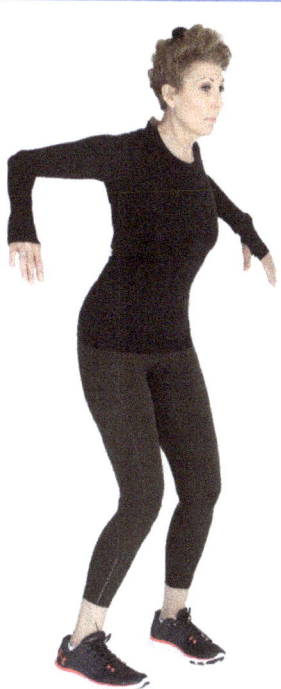

**END**

©Get Fit Gang, LLC 2020
Katie Wiseman

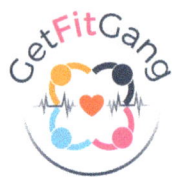

### **Modified Triceps Kickback's:** Largest muscle of the upper arm

**Set-Up:**

- Lift lightest set of weight available, 1-2 lb. and place in palms.
- If you don't have weights light enough, don't use weights and see alternate movement below.
- Lean forward with shoulders in front of hips but keeping heart and chest open. Try not to round shoulders forward, but use back muscles to keep shoulders dropped down and back (think of the pencil between the shoulder blades again). Keep spine straight and heart open.
- Place feet firmly on the ground slightly wider than shoulder width. Knees are actively bent and heels are heavy to provide a solid foundation. Play around with this set-up until you feel really grounded.
- With weights, bend elbows generously and bring as high as the horizontal plane of the shoulders, if possible.
- Wrists stay locked. Don't move them back and forth during the movement. Keep them stable throughout task.
- Visualize reaching elbows up and in toward midline of body, then stabilize them.

**Movement:**

- Elbows remain stationary as the lower arm extends the weight up and away from the elbow.
- Elbows are constantly striving to reach up and toward mid-line of body, while shoulders remained dropped down and away from ears.
- Fully extend the lower arm up and away, pause at full extension, exhale and lower the forearm and repeat.

©Get Fit Gang, LLC 2020
Katie Wiseman

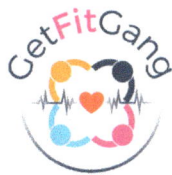

- Elbows do not move from initial position; only the lower arms moves.
- Squeeze triceps (muscles located at the back of the arm) and pause at the top of the range of movement, with elbow joint *fully* extended and exhale.
- Inhale as the weight is lowered to the shoulder. Control the weight on the way down.
- Don't swing the upper body or weights. Breath and muscles should control the weight.
- Continue, focusing on body alignment, shoulders down and away from ears, chest and heart open, elbows high and reaching toward midline, squeeze triceps at the top of the range of motion with full extension of the elbow joint, focusing on breath and a deep contraction of abdominal muscles throughout the timed task.
- Keep track from one class to the next how many repetitions you are able to accomplish. This will serve as your goal and provide incentive to grow in strength and endurance throughout the year.

**Alternate Movement (without weights)**

- Body position remains the same, but instead of bringing the lower arm in and out, keep arm fully extended behind the body above the hips.
- Raise and lower *fully* extended arms only about 1 to 2 inches, squeezing shoulder blades together and keeping chest and heart open.
- Play with palm placement. Complete 10 to 20 repetitions with palms up, repeat with palms down, and again with palms facing each other, keeping arms fully extended and as high above the hips as possible.
- Key to gaining strength is keeping arms as *long* as possible and as *high* above the hips as possible.
- Keep track from one class to the next how many long you are able to keep arms up and extended. Add weight when you feel success with this task.

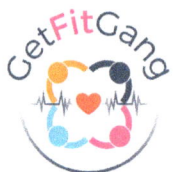

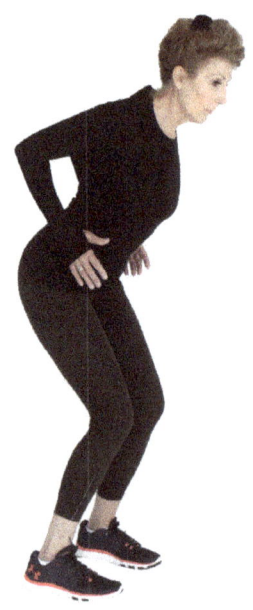

**START**

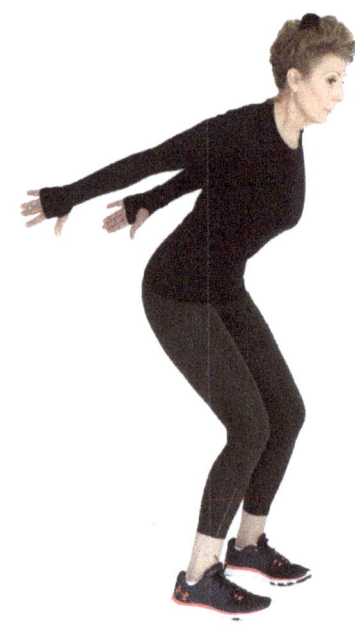

**END**

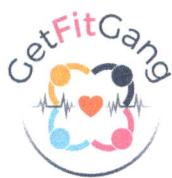

## **Modified Lunge at Steps: Targets Glutes**

Total Body Strengthener

**Set-Up:**

- Lift heaviest weights you can manage or don't use weights at all until you feel comfortable with the task.

- Place one foot onto your steps (minimum of two steps and a maximum of four) and hinge forward from the waist (Phase 1) Or, don't use the steps and simply step forward hinging chest forward (Phase 2).

- Think of tilting tailbone toward ground and hollowing out core to lengthen the lower back.

- Engage core, chest and heart open and shoulders down and away from ears.

**Movement:**

- Front foot is firmly rooted on step (or ground), with arms extended to frame each side of the leg. Shoulders are hinged forward from waist, but chest and heart are open (squeeze the shoulder blades together to open chest).

- Come up on back toes with back knee placed directly under the hip. Front knee is stacked directly over the front ankle.

- Movement is initiated by activating the core and dropping the back knee toward the floor as you remain hinged forward.

- Lower the back knee until front thigh is parallel to the floor, or as deeply as you can feeling strong and safe, then exhale as you drive *from* the front heel (key for deep glute engagement) keeping arms extended and shoulders hinged forward at the hips but heart open, to return to initial position.

- Repeat this movement pattern for 45 seconds and at half way point, switch feet.

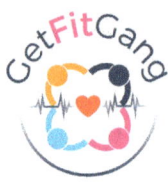

- To add a bit of challenge, pulse the back knee at the bottom of the range of movement for a set of 10-12 beats, then go back to full range for a set of 10. Repeat this series until it is time to switch legs.

- Continue, focusing on body alignment, shoulders hinged in front of hips, front knee stacked over front ankle, back knee stacked under hips, deep grounding of the front heel, exhale on the way up, inhale on the way down with a firm contraction of abdominal muscles throughout the timed task.

- Keep track from one class to the next how many repetitions you are able to accomplish. This will serve as your goal and provide incentive to grow in strength and endurance throughout the year.

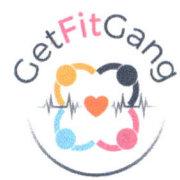

**START PHASE 1** 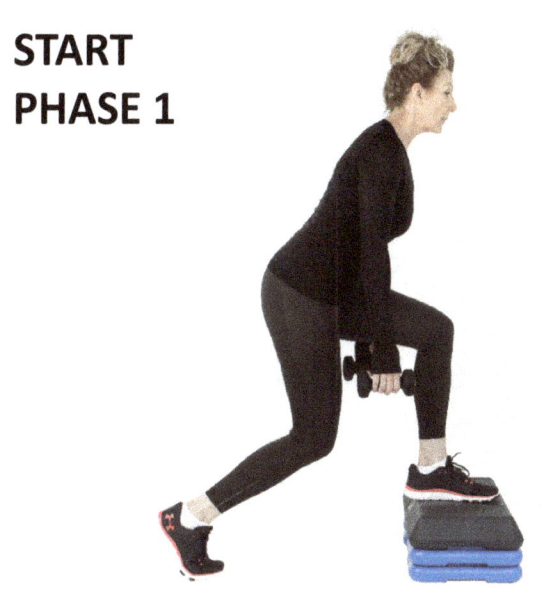 **END PHASE 1**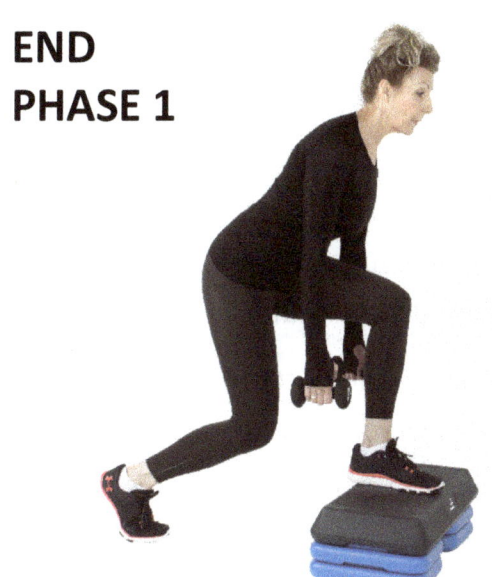

**START PHASE 2** 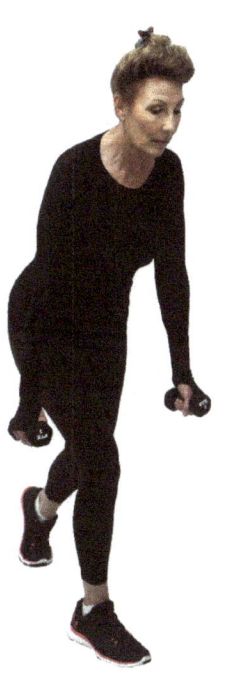 **END PHASE 2**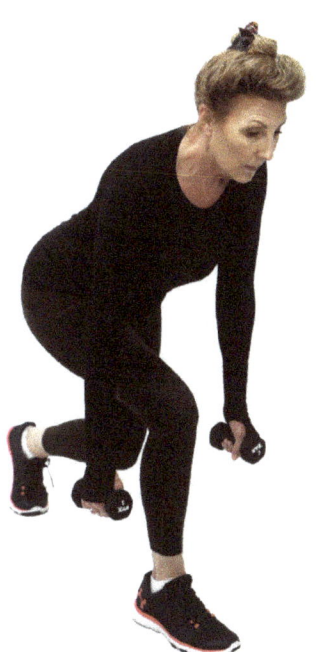

Instructional Guide Modified Tasks

©Get Fit Gang, LLC 2020
Katie Wiseman

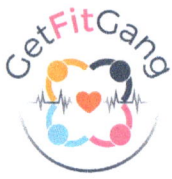

## **Modified Squat at wall with ball:** Targets Thighs and Glutes

**Total Body Strengthener**

**Set–Up:**

- Pick up 10" exercise ball and place directly behind the lower back and sandwich the ball between your back and the a wall.

- Once the ball is stabilized, walk your feet out away from the wall by pushing on the ball so once you drop your hips the knees will not fall in front of the shoe laces.

- Place weights in a chair right next to your station so you are able to reach for the weights without dislodging the ball, or moving your foot placement. You could even have someone hand you the weights.

- Knees are slightly opened with toes facing toward 11 o'clock and 1 o'clock. During movement, knees track in the same line, with the knee facing toward middle toes at the depth of movement.

- Engage core, chest and heart open and shoulders down and away from ears.

**Movement:**

- Initiate movement by engaging the core and pushing against the ball to lower the hips back and away from knees toward wall. You will notice the ball move up the spine. Push forcefully against the ball so you feel stable and the shoulders don't fall forward as the hips fall under and behind the ball.

- The weights are held in the hands extended to the side of the body.

- Lower the hips until the thighs are parallel to the ground. Try not to lean forward. Shoulders should remain stacked over hips at all times.

- Ground you weight into you heels. Don't allow body weight to transfer forward toward toes by pushing against the ball. This will protect the spine and keep weight deeply grounded in the heels.

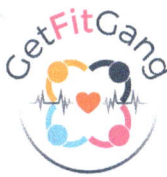

- Keep the chest lifted, heart open and core deeply engaged during the movement.

- To return to starting position, *drive* the heels into the ground as you extend the legs and bring the hips up and toward extension (keep core deeply engaged here to protect the lower back).

- Once you have reached the top of the range of motion, legs will fully extend, but the knees remain soft.

- Inhale on the way down and exhale forcefully as you drive the heels into the ground.

- Take a deep cleansing breathe at the top and repeat.

- Establish a consistent pace. Try not to rest too long at the completion of the movement. Your body craves oxygen; breathe deeply during this full body task to develop deep strength in all the major muscle groups of the body.

- Continue, focusing on body alignment, breath and a deep contraction of abdominal muscles throughout the timed task.

- Keep track from one class to the next how many repetitions you are able to accomplish. This will serve as your goal and provide incentive to grow in strength and endurance throughout the year.

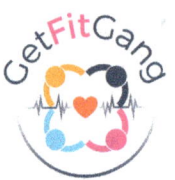

Instructional Guide Modified Tasks

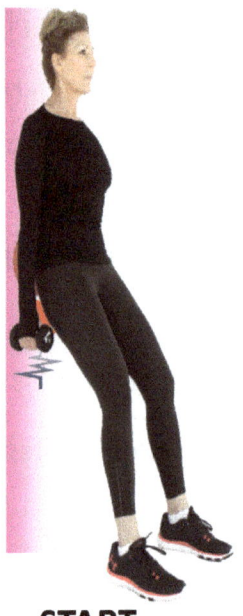

**START**

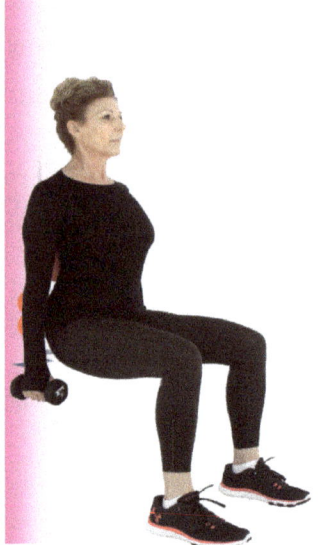

**END**

©Get Fit Gang, LLC 2020
Katie Wiseman

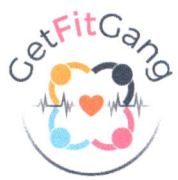

## Transition Time Chart

| Activity | Time |
|---|---|
| STEPS | 0 – 1.30 |
| Transition | :30 |
| PUSH UPS | 2:00-3:30 |
| Transition | :30 |
| ABDOMINALS | 4:00-5:30 |
| Transition | :30 |
| STEPS | 6:00-7:30 |
| Transition | :30 |
| F.A PLANK | 8:00-9:30 |
| Transition | :30 |
| GLUTE BRIDGE | 10:00-11:30 |
| Transition | :30 |
| STEPS | 12:00-13:30 |
| Transition | :30 |
| S.A. PLANK | 14:00-15:30 |
| Transition | :30 |
| SHOULDER RAISES | 16:00-17:30 |
| Transition | :30 |
| STEPS | 18:00-19:30 |
| Transition | :30 |
| REV. FLYS | 20:00-21:30 |
| Transition | :30 |
| TRICEP KICK | 22:00-23:30 |
| Transition | :30 |
| STEPS | 24:00-25:30 |
| Transition | :30 |
| LUNGE | 26:00-27:30 |
| Transition | :30 |
| SQUATS | 28:00-29:30 |
| Transition | :30 |
| STEPS | 30:00-31:30 |

| Activity | Time |
|---|---|
| STEPS | 0 – 1.30 |
| Transition | :30 |
| PUSH UPS | 2:00-3:30 |
| Transition | :30 |
| ABDOMINALS | 4:00-5:30 |
| Transition | :30 |
| STEPS | 6:00-7:30 |
| Transition | :30 |
| F.A PLANK | 8:00-9:30 |
| Transition | :30 |
| GLUTE BRIDGE | 10:00-11:30 |
| Transition | :30 |
| STEPS | 12:00-13:30 |
| Transition | :30 |
| S.A. PLANK | 14:00-15:30 |
| Transition | :30 |
| SHOULDER RAISES | 16:00-17:30 |
| Transition | :30 |
| STEPS | 18:00-19:30 |
| Transition | :30 |
| REV. FLYS | 20:00-21:30 |
| Transition | :30 |
| TRICEP KICK | 22:00-23:30 |
| Transition | :30 |
| STEPS | 24:00-25:30 |
| Transition | :30 |
| LUNGE | 26:00-27:30 |
| Transition | :30 |
| SQUATS | 28:00-29:30 |
| Transition | :30 |
| STEPS | 30:00-31:30 |

Instructional Guide Modified Tasks

©Get Fit Gang, LLC 2020
Katie Wiseman

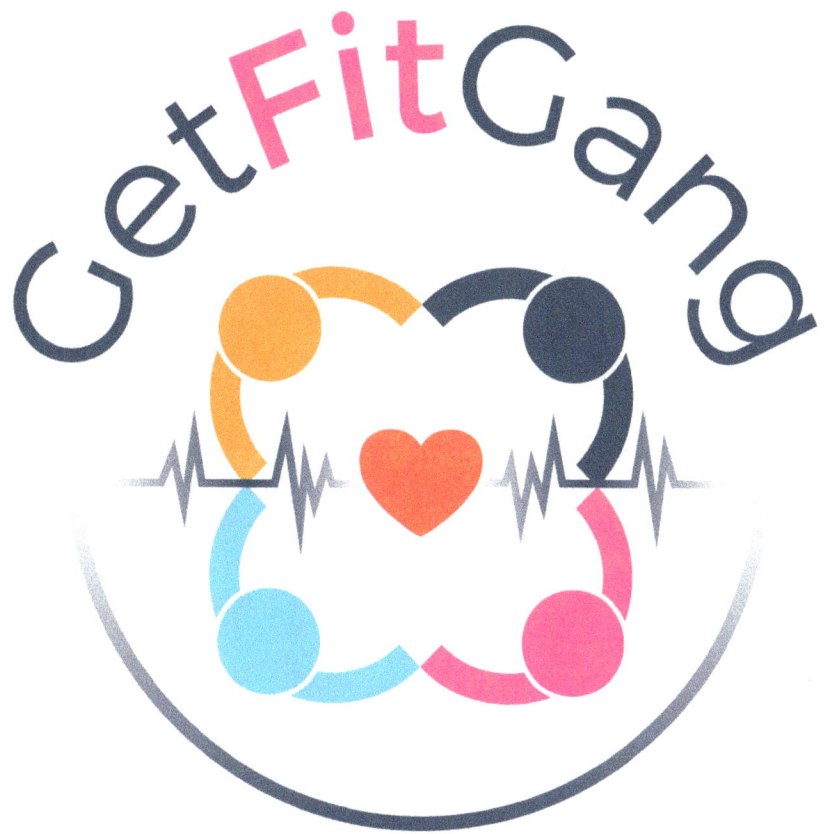

# Get Fit Gang Needed Supplies

©Get Fit Gang, LLC 2020
Katie Wiseman

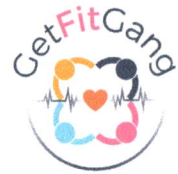

## Get Fit Gang Needed Supplies

Music, either use someone's phone or connect to Bluetooth in the gym. GFG audio or time piece.

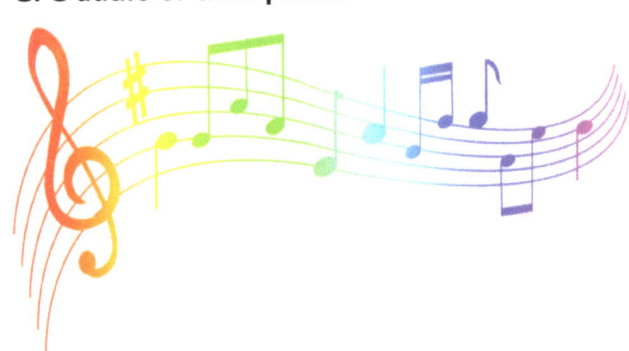

Time chart card to manage tasks.

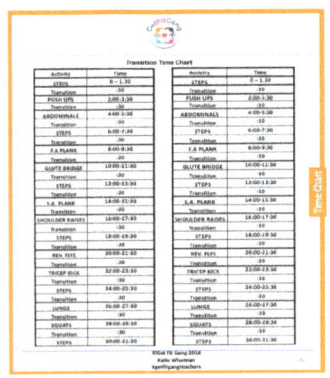

4"- 5" thick yoga mat.         or         2 large gymnastic mats.

Typically found on each campus; 2 stations per mat)

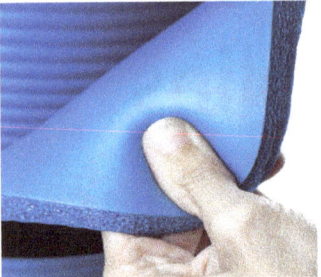
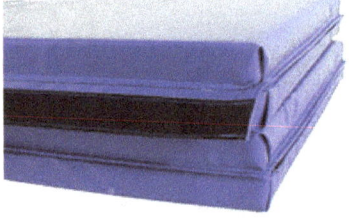

©Get Fit Gang, LLC 2020
Katie Wiseman

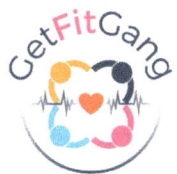

## Get Fit Gang Needed Supplies

**Steps for each Gang Member.**

(Example of steps with riser typically found at retail stores)     (Example of stackable steps typically found in schools)

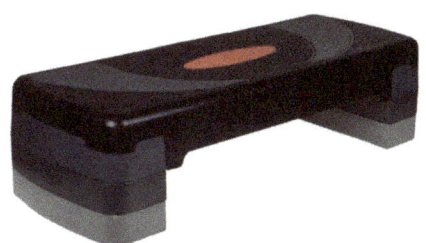  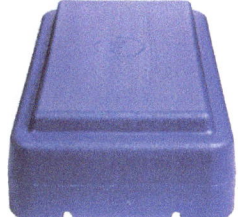

(4) 6"-8" balls set in a ring beside Abdominals, Forearm Plank, Straight Arm Plank and Modified Bridge with Ball stations.

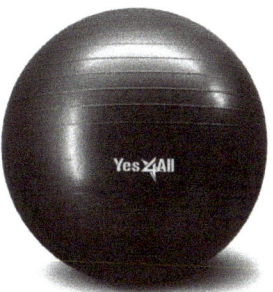

(1) - 10" – 12" ball to use for modified squat at wall.

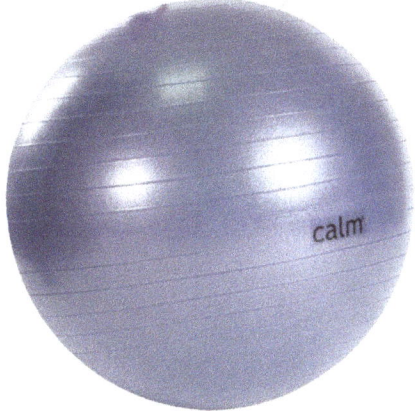

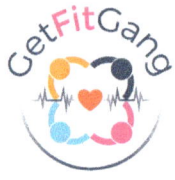

**Get Fit Gang Supplies**

**Exercise band for glutes .**

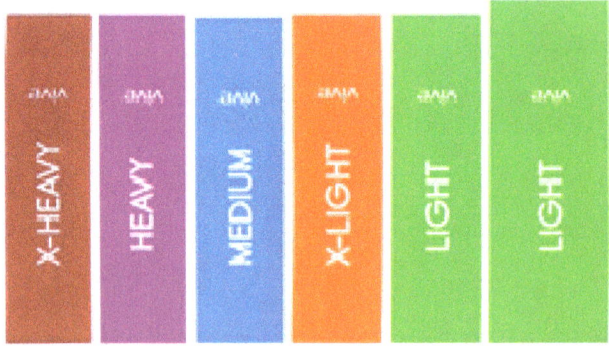

**Heavy set of weights/Light set of weights** – This may be the only equipment not typically found on a campus. But the expense is minimal. Or, perhaps you can borrow some weights.

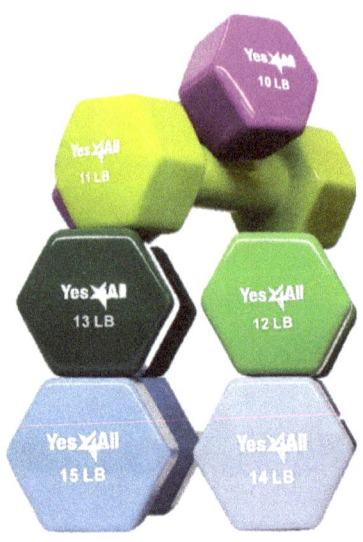
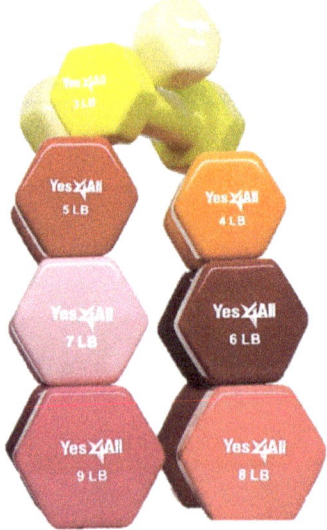

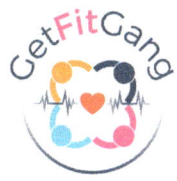

| Company | Item | Picture | Product Number | Price |
|---|---|---|---|---|
| Walmart | Everyday Essentials All-purpose ½ inch high density foam exercise mat with carrying strap. | | Walmart # 572060351 | 12.99 each |
| Walmart | CALHOME 30" Aerobic Step Aerobics Trainer Adjustable Exercise Fitness Workout Stepper | | Walmart # 565429218 | 21.79 each |
| Walmart | Valeo 9-Inch Core Training Ball, Core Training, Improves Core Strength, Balance, and Strength | | Walmart # 551490296 | 8.76 each |
| Walmart | Furinno Fitness 12-Inch LOOP Stretch Latex Exercise Band 4-PC Set | | Walmart # 566929764 | 8.99 Each |
| Walmart | XPRT Fitness 20 LB. Neoprene Dumbbell Set. 3 Pairs of Hand Weights – Home Gym workout Dumbbells. | | Walmart # 575271018 | 23.99 |
| Walmart | Neoprene Dumbbells with Non Slip Grip - Great for Total Body Workout - | | Walmart # 567245695 | 26.00 estimate |
| Total | | | | 102.52 |

Get Fit Gang Needed Supplies

©Get Fit Gang, LLC 2020
Katie Wiseman

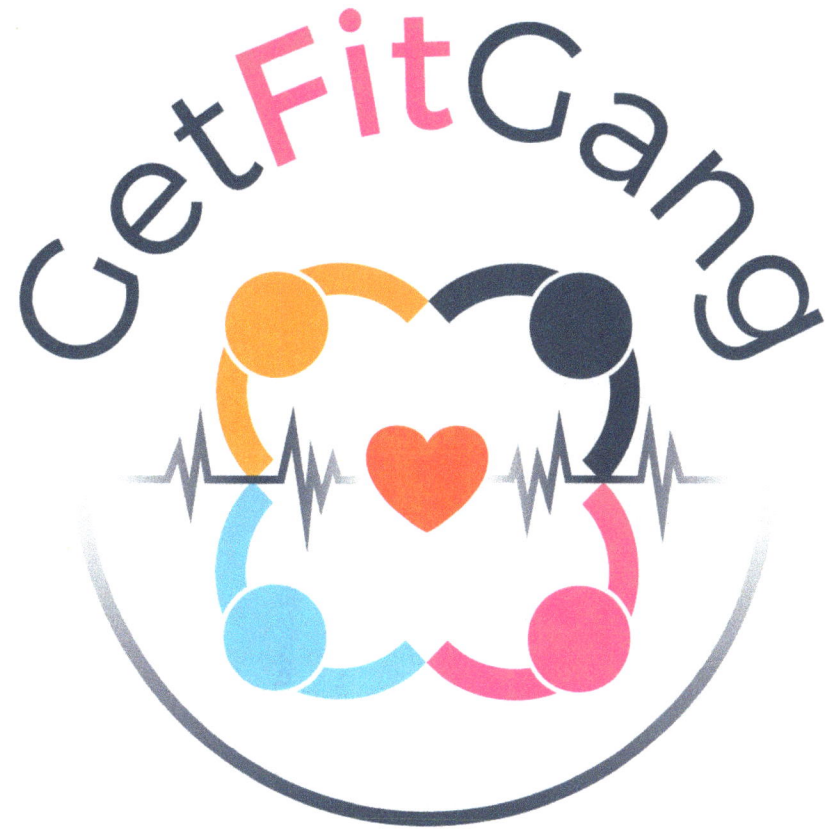

# Get Fit Gang
# Exercise Tracker Form

©Get Fit Gang, LLC 2020
Katie Wiseman

CUT ALONG THE DOTTED LINE AND AND HANG THE PERSONAL EXERCISE TRACKER IN YOUR WORKOUT SPACE

# Get Fit Gang Personal Exercise Tracker

| | | | Measurements | | |
|---|---|---|---|---|---|
| Start Date | | | | Start | End |
| End Date | | | Upper Arm | | |
| Weight | Goal | | Bust | | |
| | Start | | Waist | | |
| BMI | Goal | | Hips | | |
| | Start | End | Thighs | | |

## Get Fit Gang Sessions Attended

| January | February | March | April | May | June | July | August | September | October | November | December |
|---|---|---|---|---|---|---|---|---|---|---|---|
| 1 2 3 | 1 2 3 | 1 2 3 | 1 2 3 | 1 2 3 | 1 2 3 | 1 2 3 | 1 2 3 | 1 2 3 | 1 2 3 | 1 2 3 | 1 2 3 |
| 4 5 6 | 4 5 6 | 4 5 6 | 4 5 6 | 4 5 6 | 4 5 6 | 4 5 6 | 4 5 6 | 4 5 6 | 4 5 6 | 4 5 6 | 4 5 6 |
| 7 8 9 | 7 8 9 | 7 8 9 | 7 8 9 | 7 8 9 | 7 8 9 | 7 8 9 | 7 8 9 | 7 8 9 | 7 8 9 | 7 8 9 | 7 8 9 |
| 10 11 12 | 10 11 12 | 10 11 12 | 10 11 12 | 10 11 12 | 10 11 12 | 10 11 12 | 10 11 12 | 10 11 12 | 10 11 12 | 10 11 12 | 10 11 12 |

| Beginning Reflection | Mid Year Reflection | End Year Reflection |
|---|---|---|
| | | |

## Get Fit Gang Exercise Tracker Form

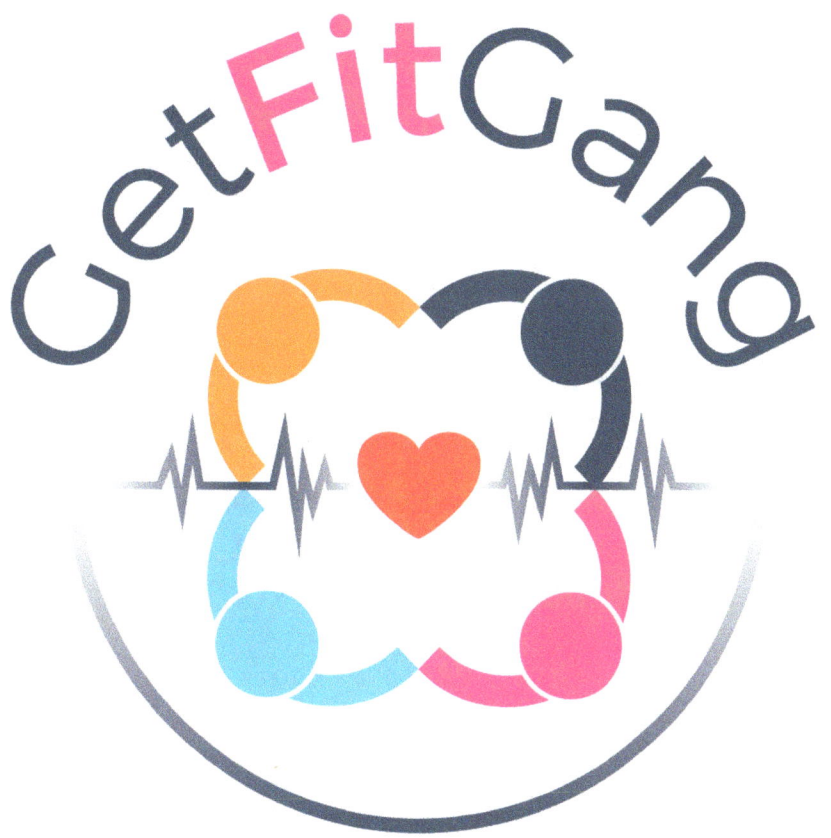

# Contact Information

©Get Fit Gang, LLC 2020
Katie Wiseman

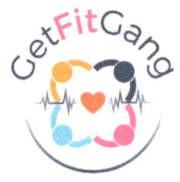

# Contact Information

Katie Wiseman

Phone Number: 713-515-3448

Website: get-fit-gang.com

Email: katie@get-fit-gang.com

Facebook
Teachers Get Fit Gang

Instagram:
@_getfitgang

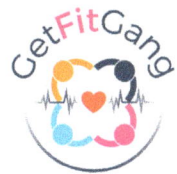

# About the Author

Katie Wiseman, a standout high school girls' basketball player received all state honors and a full scholarship to Rice University where she played Division I Women's Basketball. Upon graduation she served as the university's first graduate assistant in charge of the team's strength and conditioning program, as well as having on-the-floor coaching responsibilities.

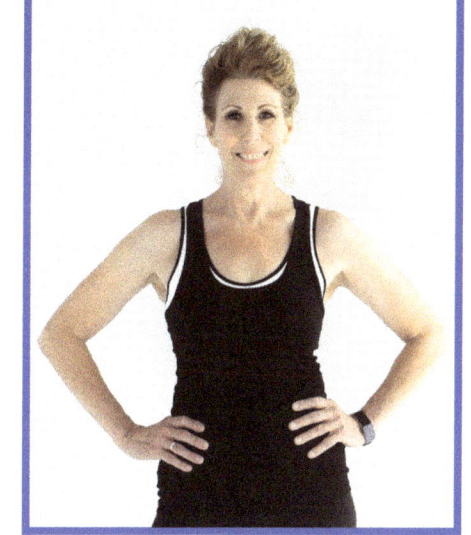

Katie earned a Master's in Teaching during her 2-year stint as a collegiate coach, whereupon she entered the high school coaching ranks for an additional three years before she took a hiatus to raise her four children. While at home with her brood, Katie received three U.S. utility patents for innovative sports training devises for young children and those with special disabilities.

She also holds a Master's degree in Educational Psychology, the field of study that focuses on the behavior of learning, and completed Texas' Administrative and Leadership certification to serve as principal of a school.

Katie has been a teacher and coach for over three decades, teaching the Get Fit Gang Fitness Program over the past 16 years. She lives in Houston, Texas and is the successful mother of four grown children who enjoys spending time practicing yoga, reading and taking the short trip down south to walk along the beach.

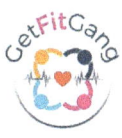

# Exercise Stations – Individual Version

## Push-Ups - Station 1

Engage Core – Drill navel to spine!
Hands wide and in alignment with shoulders.
Straighten legs behind you.
Hips in alignment with shoulders.
Inhale as you lower your chest to floor.
Exhale as you push from both hands back to starting position.
Think of yourself as a moving plank.

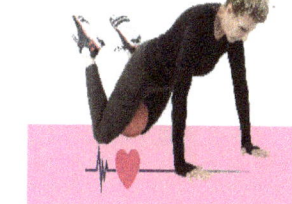

## Abdominal Curl - Station 2

Place feet on floor with hips and back on mat.
Hands under head, elbows wide to provide support to the neck.
Initiate the core and lift the shoulder blades off the mat leading with the chest,
not chin (Think apple between chin and chest).
Exhale as you squeeze the abdominals at the top of the range of motion.
Inhale on the way down and repeat.

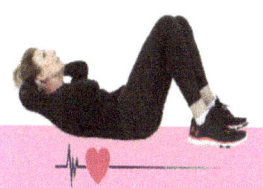

## Forearm Plank - Station 3

Extend legs behind you off the mat.
Get high on balls of the feet.
Place elbows on mat to form the number 11 (train tracks).
Lift hips to shoulder level, tighten core and stack shoulders directly over elbows.
Round out upper back by expanding the shoulder blades and dropping shoulders
    down and out.
Breathe!

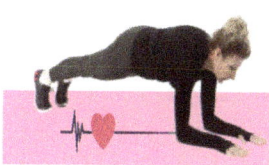

## Bridge with Band - Station 4

Place resistance band above knees. Lay down with feet off mat.
Initiate movement by engaging the core and driving your heels into the floor.
Lift hips up as far as you can without arching back, keeping shoulder blades on mat.
Squeeze the glutes at the top of the range of movement and exhale as you return
    to starting position.
Think "Up, Out, In, Down"  4 step movement!

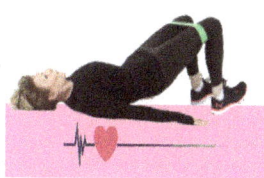

## Straight Arm Plank – Station 5

Extend legs behind you off the mat.
Get high on balls of the feet.
Place hands directly below each shoulder, with a soft bend in the elbow.
Lift hips to shoulder level, tighten core and keep shoulders stacked directly
    over wrists.
Round upper back, hollow out chest.
Keep core tight and breathe!

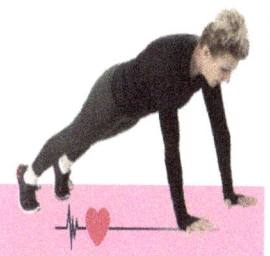

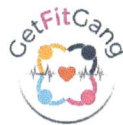

# Exercise Stations – Individual Version

### Shoulder Raises – Station 6

Core engaged.

Feet shoulder width apart, knees bent, slight tilt of the tailbone (tipped toward ground).

Keep shoulders dropped down and back, heart and chest open.

Lift weight to shoulder height (alternate front of body and side of body) keeping a soft bend in the elbow.

Exhale at the top of the movement and inhale as the weight comes down.

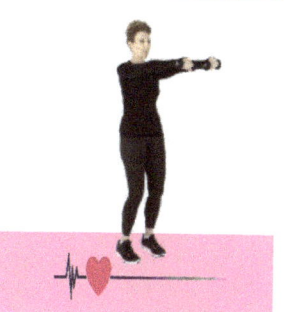

### Reverse Flys – Station 7

Engage Core.

Feet shoulder width apart, knees bent, slight tilt of the tailbone (tipped toward ground).

Hinge forward from hips, keeping shoulders down and back, heart and chest open.

Arms in the shape of a barrel. Arms keep this barrel shape as the elbows extend up and back, squeezing the shoulder blades.

Exhale at top of movement, Inhale on the way back.

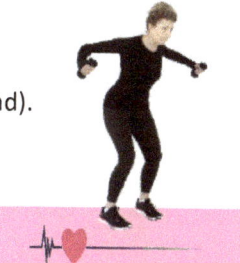

### Triceps Kickbacks - Station 8

Engage Core.

Feet shoulder width apart, knees bent, slight tilt of the tailbone (tipped toward ground).

Extend elbows high above the hips reaching up and toward the midline of the body.

Extend the weight to full extension, exhale at the top and inhale as the weights return back.

Fully extend elbow and squeeze.

Wrists stay locked.

### Lunges – Station 9

Take an extended step forward, core engaged as you drop the back knee toward the ground.

Arms are extended to the sides of the body.

Shoulders stay stacked over hips.

Keep front knee stacked over front ankle. Don't slide knee forward.

Drive the front heel into the ground, as you exhale to return to starting position.

Ideal depth front thigh parallel to ground.

### Squats – Station 10

Feet wider than shoulder width apart, toes point toward 11 o'clock and 1 o'clock.

Engage core and push hips back and away and away from feet as you bend the knees to lower the hips until thighs are parallel to ground.

Use weights or lift arms as counter balance.

Exhale and drive your heels into the ground as you lift the hips and extend the thighs to starting position.

Inhale and repeat.

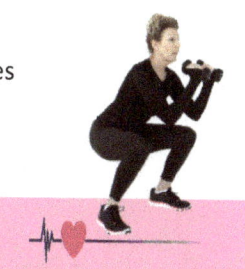

www.ingramcontent.com/pod-product-compliance
Lightning Source LLC
Chambersburg PA
CBHW081200020426
42333CB00020B/2575